Rebel
Homemaker

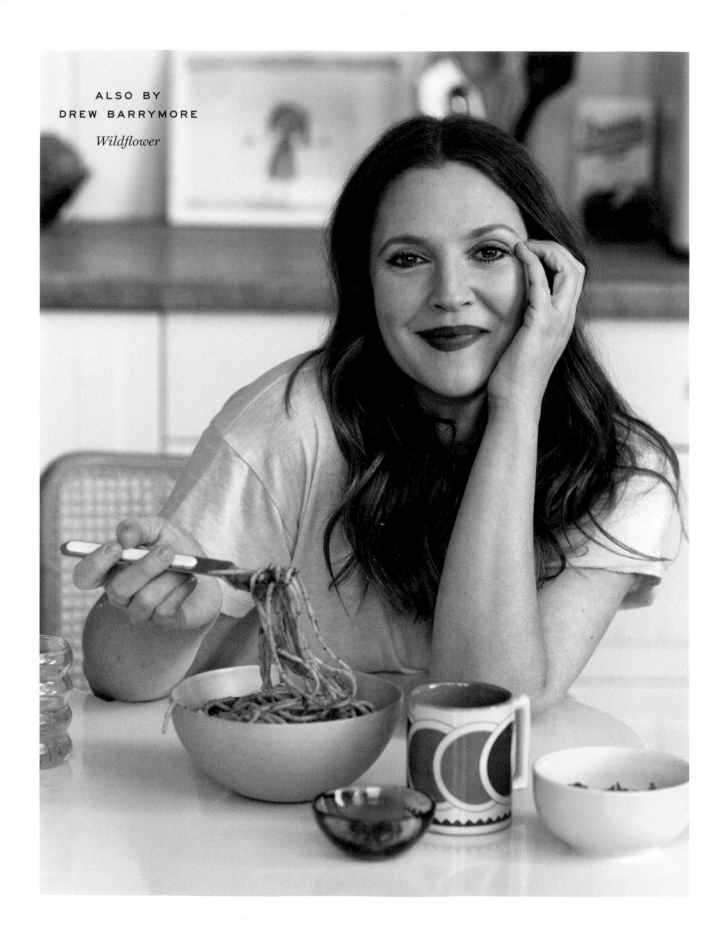

ALSO BY
DREW BARRYMORE

Wildflower

Rebel Homemaker

FOOD

~

FAMILY

~

LIFE

DREW BARRYMORE

with Pilar Valdes

DUTTON

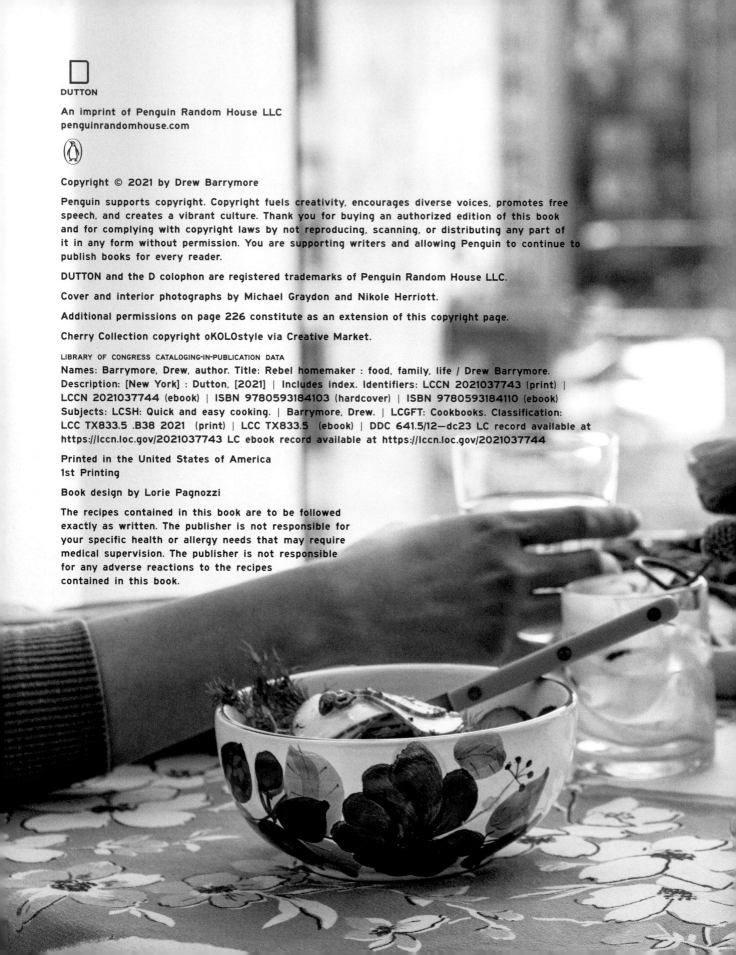

DUTTON

An imprint of Penguin Random House LLC
penguinrandomhouse.com

Cover and interior photographs by Michael Graydon and Nikole Herriott.

Additional permissions on page 226 constitute as an extension of this copyright page.

Cherry Collection copyright oKOLOstyle via Creative Market.

LIBRARY OF CONGRESS CATALOGING-IN-PUBLICATION DATA
Names: Barrymore, Drew, author. Title: Rebel homemaker : food, family, life / Drew Barrymore. Description: [New York] : Dutton, [2021] | Includes index. Identifiers: LCCN 2021037743 (print) | LCCN 2021037744 (ebook) | ISBN 9780593184103 (hardcover) | ISBN 9780593184110 (ebook) Subjects: LCSH: Quick and easy cooking. | Barrymore, Drew. | LCGFT: Cookbooks. Classification: LCC TX833.5 .B38 2021 (print) | LCC TX833.5 (ebook) | DDC 641.5/12—dc23 LC record available at https://lccn.loc.gov/2021037743 LC ebook record available at https://lccn.loc.gov/2021037744

Printed in the United States of America
1st Printing

Book design by Lorie Pagnozzi

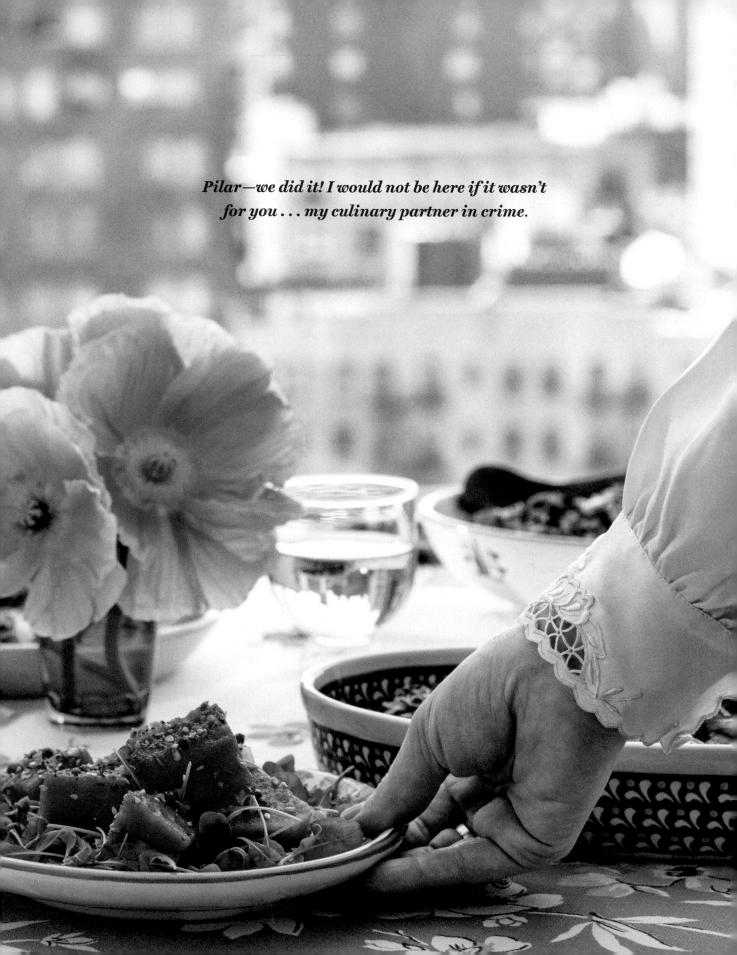

*Pilar—we did it! I would not be here if it wasn't
for you . . . my culinary partner in crime.*

Contents

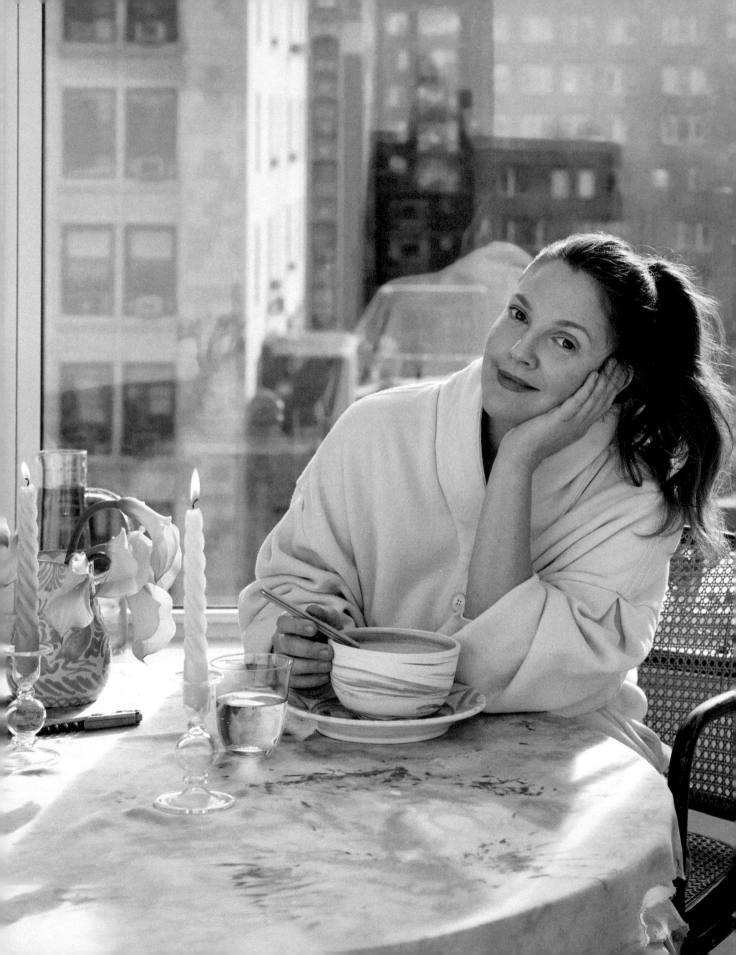

Introduction

I love . . .

Honey

Cumin

Saffron

Cracked black pepper

I hate . . .

Truffles

Goat cheese

Lamb

I love cookbooks

I collect cookbooks

I love reading cookbooks

I love ordering cookbooks

I love shopping for cookbooks

I love cooking from cookbooks

My cookbooks have come with me from one home to another

I've learned to dog-ear the pages instead of sticking Post-its everywhere

I can recognize a cookbook wherever I go

And I think every cookbook has *one* recipe that will change your life!

I love creamy pasta

I love making soups

I am a one-pot girl

Multitasking, I'm a bit screwed

I can't cook for large groups

I'm a personal chef

I like to cook for myself without judgment

Why do so many recipes have to be for four to six?

Solo by Anita Lo helps

My home is a test kitchen

We are *always* cooking

Pilar Valdes and I are always deconstructing food

Figuring out new ways to make things in healthy ways

But we also love the classics

Our mission is to have two options:

The most decadent one and the most conscious dish as well

For those fortunate enough to have food right now . . .

I have heard comfort food is through the roof

Everyone is trying to soothe

Food . . .

I think of chefs as rock stars

I geek out

But I've learned in this unprecedented time

That those who work in food banks are superheroes

They deserve all the support and the cheers and the donations and the attention

That said . . .

Next in line for superhero:

Grocery store workers and food deliverers!

I love that they are our heroes!

The people providing food on the front lines

I love food

I appreciate food

And those who provide it

I don't take any of it for granted

And anytime I am in need of comfort

I turn to

Kraft Macaroni & Cheese

DELUXE

Not powder

With cracked black pepper

And *Dumb and Dumber*

This will always make me happy

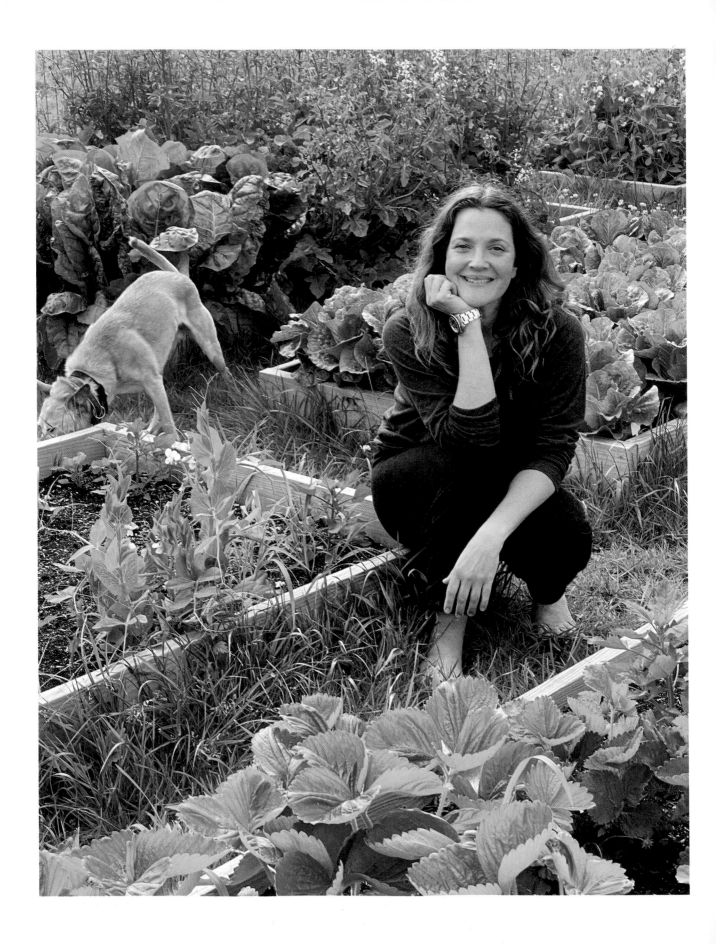

I Am Writing

Spring 2020

Everyone has been affected by the pandemic. It's been an opportunity for a world-wide reset. The questions that burn in my mind are these: If we are forced to live differently, can we be inspired to think differently? Is this when Zoom conferencing and workout streaming become the norm? Is this when we recognize what we do and don't need? Is this when we go back to pioneering a healthier way of life? Imagine if we didn't travel so much. I can't begin to tell you how often I have to travel for meetings around the world. I love seeing the world, but flying can be stressful and is bad for the earth. I would be willing to give that up for a better, cleaner world. What if we only flew when absolutely necessary? What if we considered more than just our job or our vacation before we booked that next trip? I am self-taught, and the two ways I've learned are by reading and traveling—the two things that have made me who I am. (I think my endgame in life is to work at a travel magazine . . .) But we can all be more conscientious in our choices. Please don't get mad at me for

And this is what I have for today. I don't know how I will feel tomorrow.

suggesting "less of everything": less movement, less stress. We are literally being forced to be still right now. Forced to stay at home. None of us could have predicted we would see this in our lifetime. And yet, I can see the future. A brighter future that exists for our kids—whether they're our own kids or not.

I've always been the kind of person who hates soapboxes, and I don't mean to be up on one now. Growing up in Hollywood, I felt the sting when listening to privileged people talk about others' needs, and I especially hated it if they used their platform to take others down. I march in the army of optimism, and I've always refused to condescend or speak out negatively. There have been so many humans who have used their voices around the world to change it for the better. Maybe it's their tone? Maybe if it feels inspiring and personal instead of righteous? Is that the secret sauce for humans from anywhere and everywhere daring to speak up? After all, it's always been humans who have inspired us. Therefore, everyone has the potential to be someone who will change the world in big and small ways.

What are people thinking right now? What inventions and ideas and new ways of doing things are being thought up in the face of this crisis? What will be the outcome? The innovations? If we make it through this, and I know we will, I almost hope people don't overindulge in the return to life as it was before. Life moving forward should be altered. Wouldn't it be great to live differently? Think differently? Work differently?

I myself have put my shiny tech things down and picked up writing. My business partner Nancy Juvonen always tells me, no matter what I am going through in life, I

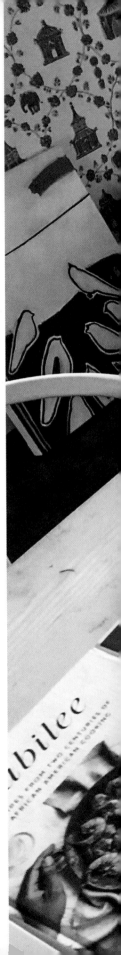

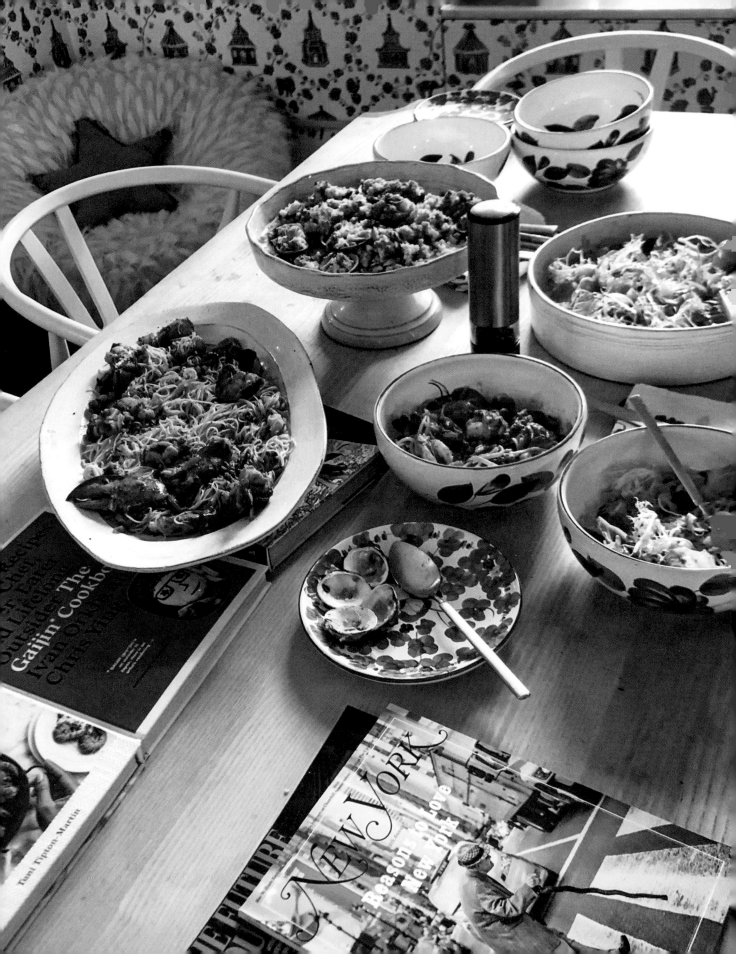

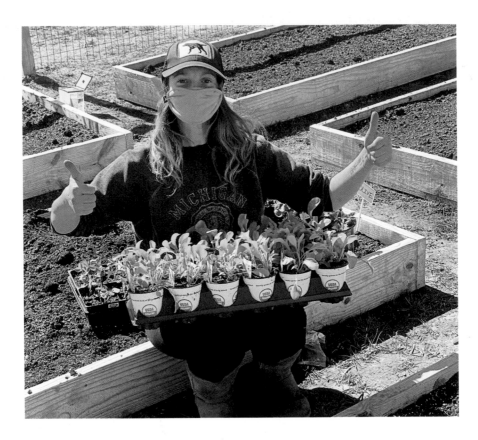

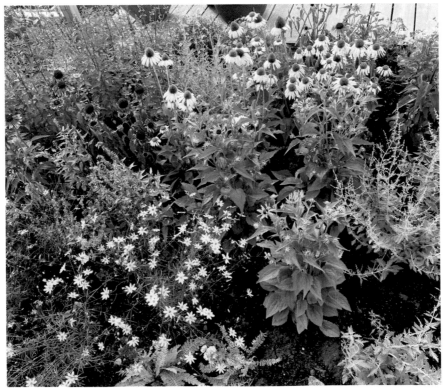

should write. Heartbreak? Write. Lost? Write. Need to communicate with someone in a deeper way? Write! How about the way we communicate with ourselves? I was so lost after giving birth the first time. I was bent so out of shape the first few days I thought I would die of fear. I couldn't sleep or eat and I was becoming incapable of thinking straight. And then a package came to my door from a dear friend. It was a journal with small daily spaces to fill. Not overwhelming. And so I started writing to my daughter. I would say in a few sentences what the day brought. I wrote in it every day for three years. I plan to give it to her when she is eighteen, ten years from now.

What if we all just started journaling a few sentences of this journey? I always talk about collective experiences. This is a time when everyone is in the same boat. Staying home. Living in this wild and terrifying time of struggle is our new normal. Great art and community can come out of the most difficult times. Change comes from times like this. Change in perception and behavior. I invite us all to write a few sentences every day. And we will be able to look back when we are all older and see what this time actually was… is. But that is a small and personal idea. How we take care of each other in this moment obviously comes first. Empathy has never been more important. Maybe we're supposed to take care of everyone and everything and have this newfound humility and respect for our surroundings. This is a health crisis that affects everyone—the entire planet is involved. And we can't go back or ignore what is happening, and maybe this is a sign that not only do we need to save our planet but also we need to save ourselves. I think humans thrive the most when we take care of each other. And if there is a way to empower ourselves without being selfish and heal our planet without being political, just a nurturing and cultivating of our world and our lives, then we can all thrive. Humans don't take things lying down. We are proactive and inventive. I cannot wait to see the good that comes out of this. Yes, I march in the army of optimism, and while we might be marching in place for a while, it's okay if we fall apart and put ourselves back

I will look for that infallible hope I own, and harness it.

together. This will be ongoing. And this is what I have for today. I don't know how I will feel tomorrow. I don't know what will happen tomorrow. Maybe this whole thing I have written will seem beyond trivial. I am just writing with my heart and my hope. And maybe I will have even more words to illustrate life to my daughters one day.

By the way, we bought six chicks (talk about going back to the old ways). We're gonna have eggs. I am going to kiss my kids. I'm going to pray for healthcare workers. I'm going to try not to burst into tears as my TV tells me things are getting worse. I am going to help my friend Kate with a way to donate money. I'm gonna look at the baby chickens and marvel at their cuteness. I'm going to do as much as I can today to stay hopeful, knowing I am going to fall hard and have to dust myself off again. I am going to be grateful to all of those people who are not overthinking everything they say or do. I am going to feel insecure about sharing this. I'm going to wipe the tears that are streaming down my face right now and then freak out about touching my face. I'm going to lose hope. And then I am going to reread what I wrote and realize that I was optimistic and problem-solving when I began to write. Because it's there. It's there to look back on. And since no one can travel the world right now, I will hold on to reading and writing. And then maybe a little escape viewing later. Thank God for all the creators who help us get a little lost right now. Thank God for all those who help us get found, too.

I am finding my words. Wobbly one minute. Full of conviction the next. But I am daring to put this into words. And just for today, I am grateful. The way I hope to be. Grateful for everything I have gotten to do. Grateful for my daughters. Grateful for my laptop. Grateful to know when to turn off the news. Grateful to go and search for bits of wisdom rather than twenty-four-hour doom cycles. I am going to look within and go find that place inside that feels strong. That problem-solves. That believes in the high road. That knows my place in the universe. The place where I believe that something wonderful will come out of this. A worldwide reset. It will not be easy. But it's in motion. And hopefully, in the best way possible, the world will never be the same. But also hopefully, the world will be new. That is what a reset is: it takes everything away, and we start over. Stronger and smarter. I will go back to my earlier sentence. I cannot wait to see what comes out of this. And as soon as I can, I will figure out how to get dye, because the girls want to tie-dye. And tonight the world will be full of Zoom chats and quiet moments, too, as we go back to our own private worlds. I will look for that infallible hope I own, and I will harness it.

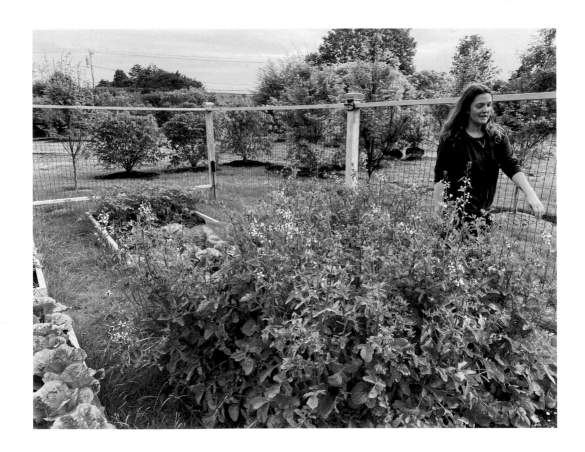

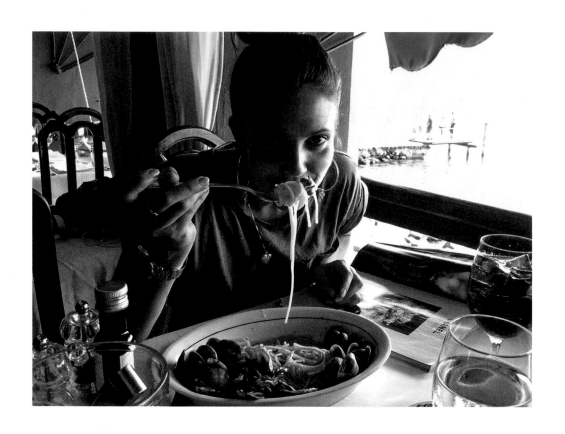

Thirty Meals of a Lifetime

1. Definitely in a cave in Italy, on Lake Garda, where I ate spaghetti vongole. I still have a picture of it I keep on my desk.

2. It wasn't eating, but it was drinking Tusker beers with a bunch of gentlemen at a refugee camp in Africa. It was raining giant bugs from the trees above, all over us, as the sun set. And it was a great moment, and gathering, that I'll never forget.

3. Getting the pleasure of having the dish famously called Oysters and Pearls by French Laundry's chef, Thomas Keller. It is simply one oyster with caviar and some viscous sauce that brings the whole thing together and explodes in your mouth like the most decadent bite you've ever taken in your life.

4. Dinner at the bar at Osteria Mozza, Nancy Silverton's restaurant, eating prosciutto di parma and figs and thinking I had died and gone to heaven.

5. My mom's tuna noodle casserole.

6. Japanese breakfast at the Park Hyatt Tokyo, looking out the glass windows at the city. It was a perfect little salmon, the sweet delicious sushi rice, the spinach, the egg, the miso broth steaming with fresh herbs. Japanese breakfast is my absolute favorite.

7. Eating a box of Kraft Macaroni & Cheese with lots of cracked pepper and a giant bottle of red wine, crying to *Sex and the City* after my boyfriend broke up with me.

8. Eating in Bangkok at a hotel that had the best Thai food of my life. My friend got so red in the face from all the spices, and we laughed and laughed, and we ate right on the river. I love Thai food—I've eaten a lot of it in my life—but this was simply the Mount Everest of Thai cuisine experiences.

9. Getting to eat with the famous Jiro in his underground sushi restaurant in the subway station in Tokyo. There is a documentary made about this man, who is a genius and a master at his art, and I actually got to eat his food! And totally got a picture to prove it.

10. Driving through the In-N-Out Burger drive-through in California. You'll never have a better cheeseburger in your life.

11. I went to Santa Fe for four days and every single morning I ate at the same restaurant I found there. I still have the cookbook! It was lively, cozy, and the food was incredible. All of their flavors were so powerful.

12. Black-Eyed Susan's in Nantucket. They have an egg scramble with Thai green curry and chopped-up broccoli that's the greatest breakfast in the world. It's in this hot, tiny joint with no fans and a flat-top grill and wood paneling. And there's always an hour-long wait outside.

13. Eating Joe's Pizza from New York in a cardboard box outside of a movie theater. There's nothing like 'za on a street corner, the concrete under your butt, the grease on your fingers, and the best slice of pizza there is in this country.

14. The restaurant inside the Mandarin Oriental hotel in Honolulu. We would order a bowl of vinegar sushi rice topped with grilled marinated steak, and then topped with crispy thin onion rings. We would pour extra vinegar and soy sauce all over the whole thing and just go to town. We ate this every night for three months straight while we were filming *50 First Dates*.

15. Every food truck breakfast burrito from every film that I've ever been on. I get the same thing—jack cheese, spinach, mushrooms, and egg with a side of hot sauce. Breakfast of champions!

16. Pilar's Stovetop Scampi. The first time I ever had it, it literally blew my mind. Scampi is one of my favorite dishes and I've eaten it all over the world. But not until I had Pilar's did I find my very favorite one on planet Earth. And fun fact—the recipe is in this book (page 193)!

17. Okay, bourgie—best dinner ever goes to Caviar Kaspia, and none other, in the heart of Paris. I ate a baked potato that had been slathered with massive amounts of butter and then topped with a tablespoon of caviar and I remember thinking that *this* is living. Bucket list checked.

18. A home-cooked meal in India, right in New Delhi, by the beautiful Shantum Seth. He and his family cooked me multiple dishes that were as spiritual as you can imagine.

19. In the Dominican Republic, I was staying at a hotel, and around the corner on the beach was a gathering of multiple tents that were patched together with locals cooking various dishes. It was something you couldn't even find in a guidebook because it was so low-key. This was the kind of experience that you could've only come upon by chance; no one could've told you about something so discreet. And the ceviche and the rice and the flavors . . . It was definitely one of the best meals I've ever had in my life, sitting right on plastic chairs at the folding tables they had set out. Oh, did I mention it was also raining? Pouring down, yet it was the perfect addition to the experience.

20. Drinking a Himalayan burnt sea salt margarita—and then they threw in crunchy crickets. I was like, "Um, hell no. No thank you." But I ended up eating like fifty. Turns out they really are delicious.

21. Dan Tana's in West Hollywood. It used to be called the Tana Salad, although now it's called Chopped à la Nicky Hilton. It's the greatest salad ever—chunks of iceberg, cubes of mozzarella, crunchy green bell pepper, garbanzo beans, and the best vinaigrette you've ever had in your life.

22. Lucy's El Adobe Cafe, circa the late 1970s and '80s. Lucy's was the hip Hollywood joint across from Paramount Studios. Now it's slathered with eight-by-tens of all the famous people who have eaten there over the years. Lucy had a secret garlic salad dressing and she refused to give the recipe. It's still to this day the best salad dressing I've ever had.

23. My fortieth dinner party inside my living room, with tables filled with all the people I've known my whole life, catered by Suzanne Goin. We had fried chicken, and it was like my own personal wedding.

24. Lunch at the Breakers in Australia, overlooking the big pool that meets the ocean and the rocks, and the surfers on the waves and on the beach, and it's just everything you want it to be. Seafood, ocean, glass walls, and everybody is drinking wine.

25. La Colombe d'Or Hotel in the south of France, which is famous for all the artists who have stayed there in the past 150 years and left priceless pieces on all the walls to pay for their stays. There is a restaurant in the courtyard that is laden with draping trees and branches canopied all above your head. They were wrapped in Christmas lights they'd turn on at night. I don't even remember exactly what I ate; I just remember thinking this is going to be one of my favorite meals of my entire life because of the dreamy setting.

26. A hot bowl of clam chowder upstairs in a restaurant at Pike Place Market in Seattle with tons of Tabasco and crunchy oyster crackers and cracked black pepper. I also had that same revelation at a Legal Sea Foods in the Boston airport, that it might be the best bowl of clam chowder I've ever had in my life. I love clam chowder, New England style.

27. I had paella somewhere in Amsterdam in a dark wood bar and restaurant, and it came in the giant pan, a cast-iron deal, and it really blew my doors off as the best paella!

28. A fish taco truck on Anini Beach in Kauai. It literally had a surfboard on the back that said FISH TACOS and they were the best things I've ever, ever had. You ate them under trees, right on the beach.

29. Rocky Toto's in New York, with this insane chef who would serve all different variations of beef in the most extreme and unique ways inside of that old office with wine bottles everywhere and folding tables.

30. Any breakfast my daughters make me. With varying degrees of edibility.

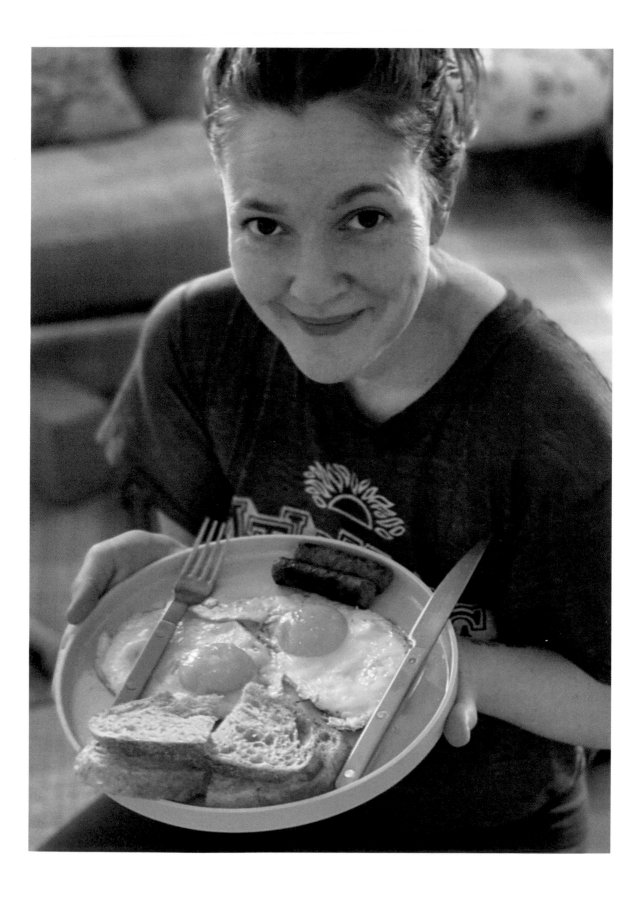

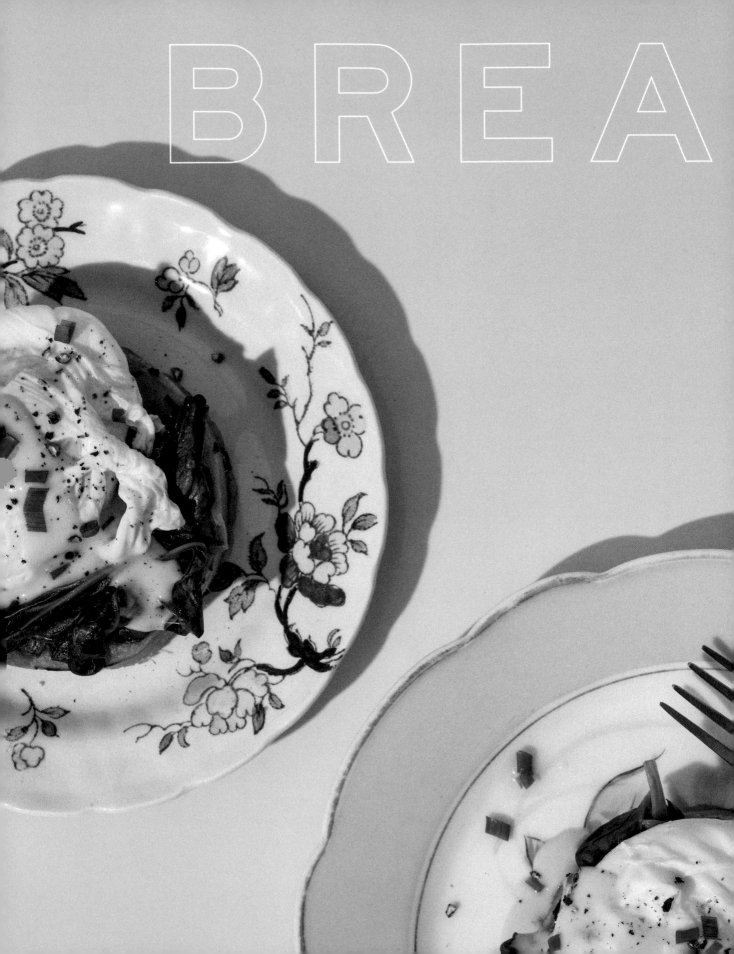

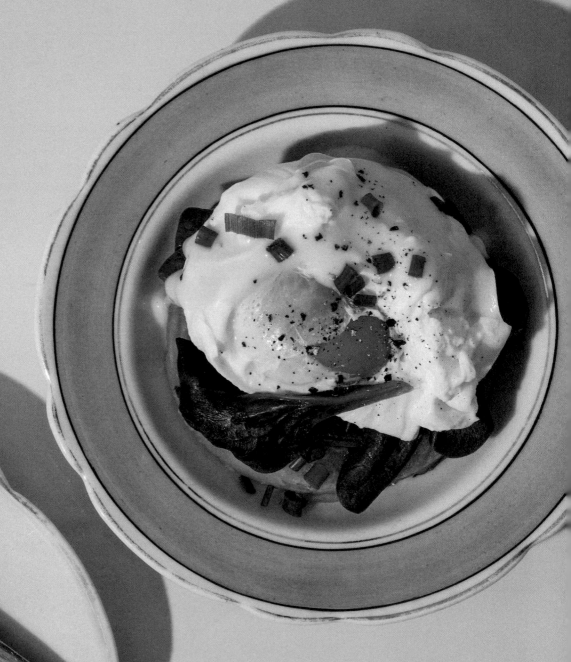

KFAST

SWEET POTATO FLORENTINE | *see page 22*

Sweet Potato Florentine

2 medium Japanese sweet
potatoes scrubbed clean,
about 1 to 1½ pounds

Kosher salt and freshly
ground black pepper

4 large eggs, plus 2 large
egg yolks, divided

1 teaspoon dijon mustard

2 teaspoons freshly
squeezed lemon juice

4 tablespoons vegan butter
or unsalted butter, melted

1 small bunch flat-leaf
spinach, stemmed, washed,
and lightly shaken dry

1 tablespoon chopped chives,
for serving

When I'm laying off the bread, these twice-cooked sweet potatoes help satisfy my brunch cravings. This dish is a cross between eggs benedict (the hollandaise) and a Florentine (the spinach), and is 100 percent delicious.

Sweet potatoes are packed with nutrients, vitamins, and fiber and are a great, affordable staple in the kitchen. We like to roast off a big batch and have them on hand to incorporate into different dishes throughout the week *(in veggie burgers! glazed in miso! in quinoa salad!)*. One of our favorite ways to use them is as a base in this Sweet Potato Florentine. We love using Japanese sweet potatoes, which we find are denser and creamier than other sweet potatoes; they also brown and crisp up nicely, which is exactly what we are looking for in this recipe.

Both the sweet potatoes and the poached eggs (yep, you read that right!) can be made in advance.

Roast the potatoes. Preheat the oven to 400 degrees. Prick the sweet potatoes all over with a fork and wrap individually with a piece of tinfoil. Roast the potatoes until very tender, 55 to 65 minutes. Unwrap and let them sit until cool enough to handle. Peel and transfer the flesh to a bowl. Mash the flesh until nearly smooth and season to taste with salt and pepper. You should have about 2 cups of mashed sweet potatoes. (This step can be done up to 5 days in advance.)

Form and bake the base. Raise the oven temperature to 425 degrees. On a baking sheet lined with parchment paper, form the sweet potato bases. Using a 3-inch ring mold or a ½-cup measuring cup, make 4 sweet potato rounds, about 3 inches wide and 1 inch high. Bake the rounds until the edges and undersides are lightly golden and crisp, 15 minutes. Set aside and keep warm.

Make the immersion blender hollandaise. Place the egg yolks, mustard, and lemon juice in a 2-cup measuring cup. Use an immersion blender to mix until frothy. Slowly drizzle in the melted butter, moving the blender up and down to help incorporate air. Continue blending until the mixture is whipped and emulsified. Season to taste with salt and pepper and keep warm. (Hollandaise can sit in the measuring cup in a small pot of warm water until ready to serve. If the sauce becomes too thick, thin with ¼ to ½ teaspoon hot water.)

Poach the eggs. Bring a medium pot of water to a boil over high heat. Reduce the heat to maintain a bare simmer, with just the smallest of bubbles rising to the top. Working one egg at a time, crack the egg into a small bowl and gently tip into the water; repeat with the remaining eggs. Let poach, undisturbed, until the whites are just set, 3 to 3½ minutes. Use a slotted spoon to remove the eggs to a paper towel–lined plate. (Do-ahead tip: poach your eggs following the instructions above and transfer the finished poached eggs into an airtight container with cold water and refrigerate. They can be made one day in advance. Just before serving, submerge the eggs into hot water for 1 minute to rewarm.)

Steam spinach. Right before serving, heat a large skillet over high heat. Add the spinach and season with salt and pepper. Cook until just wilted, stirring occasionally, about 30 seconds. Immediately transfer to a plate to prevent oversteaming.

Assemble. Divide the sweet potato rounds among serving plates. Top with steamed spinach and place a poached egg in the center. Drizzle with hollandaise, season with salt and pepper, and sprinkle with chives. Serve warm.

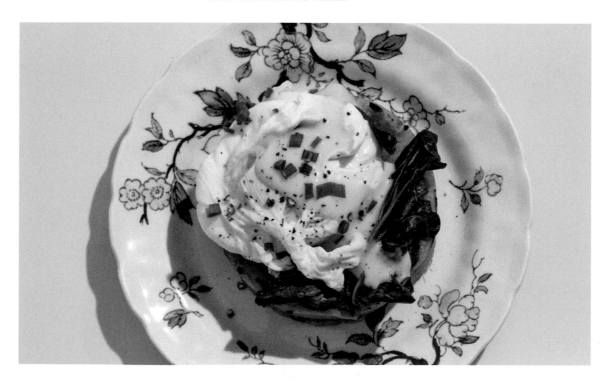

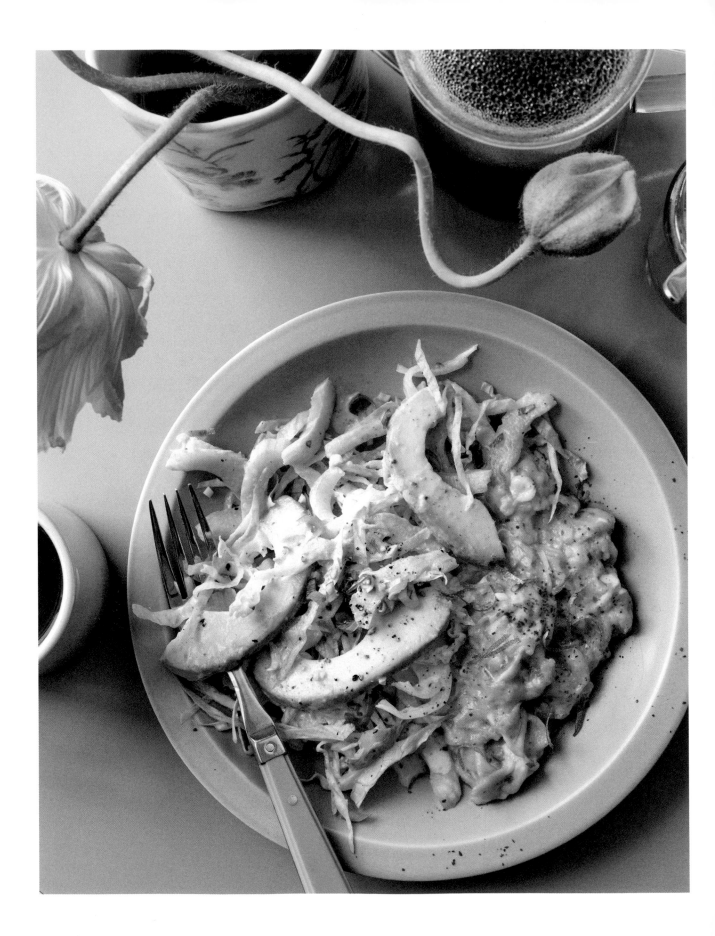

Soft-Scrambled Yuzu Kosho Eggs with Crisp Avocado Salad

SERVES 1

For the Crisp Avocado Salad

2 teaspoons of your favorite mayonnaise (I love Vegenaise for this)

1 tablespoon freshly squeezed lime juice

1 scallion, thinly sliced, white and light green parts only

½ teaspoon Sriracha, or to taste

Kosher salt and freshly ground black pepper

1 heaping cup thinly sliced iceberg lettuce

1 stalk celery, peeled and thinly sliced crosswise

½ avocado, peeled, pitted, and sliced lengthwise into ½-inch slices

For the Eggs

2 large eggs

Lime zest

½ teaspoon yuzu kosho

2 teaspoons avocado oil

Togarashi, to taste, for serving

Flaky sea salt (we love Maldon), for serving

Yuzu kosho is probably one of my favorite pantry staples, and if you haven't had it yet, Pilar and I encourage you to make room for it in your pantry pantheon! A Japanese condiment made from fresh chilies, salt, and the zest of yuzu citrus—it's the perfect combo of heat, salt, and acid that adds so much pop to dishes. It's crazy versatile and can be used with so many things from fish to vegetables to noodles—and in this case, with our soft scrambled eggs. (Just keep in mind: a little goes a long way!)

I like to have side salads with breakfast to get those greens and vegetables in first thing in the morning. This avocado salad, which is loaded with celery and iceberg lettuce, offers a wonderful textural contrast to the creamy, soft eggs. (Feel free to use your mayonnaise of choice.) Breakfast of champions, indeed.

Make the salad. In a medium bowl, combine the mayonnaise, lime juice, scallions, and sriracha. Whisk until incorporated and season to taste with salt and pepper. Add the lettuce, celery, and avocado. Gently toss to dress. Place in the refrigerator until ready to serve.

Prepare the eggs. In a small bowl, combine the eggs, lime zest, and yuzu kosho. Whisk until the mixture is homogenous and slightly frothy. (We don't season our eggs here because yuzu kosho already packs a punch of salt and heat.)

Cook the eggs. Heat the oil in a small nonstick skillet over medium heat. Pour the egg mixture into the skillet and let it set for several seconds without disturbing. Then, using a rubber spatula, begin slowly stirring and scraping the bottom and sides of the pan in a continuous motion, making sure that all the areas are cooking slowly and evenly, about 1 minute. Remove the pan from the heat right before the eggs are fully set and stir gently a few more times; the residual heat will continue to cook the eggs. The scramble should look nearly wet and have the texture of small curds.

Assemble. Transfer the eggs to a plate and garnish with togarashi and flaky sea salt. Serve immediately with the Crisp Avocado Salad.

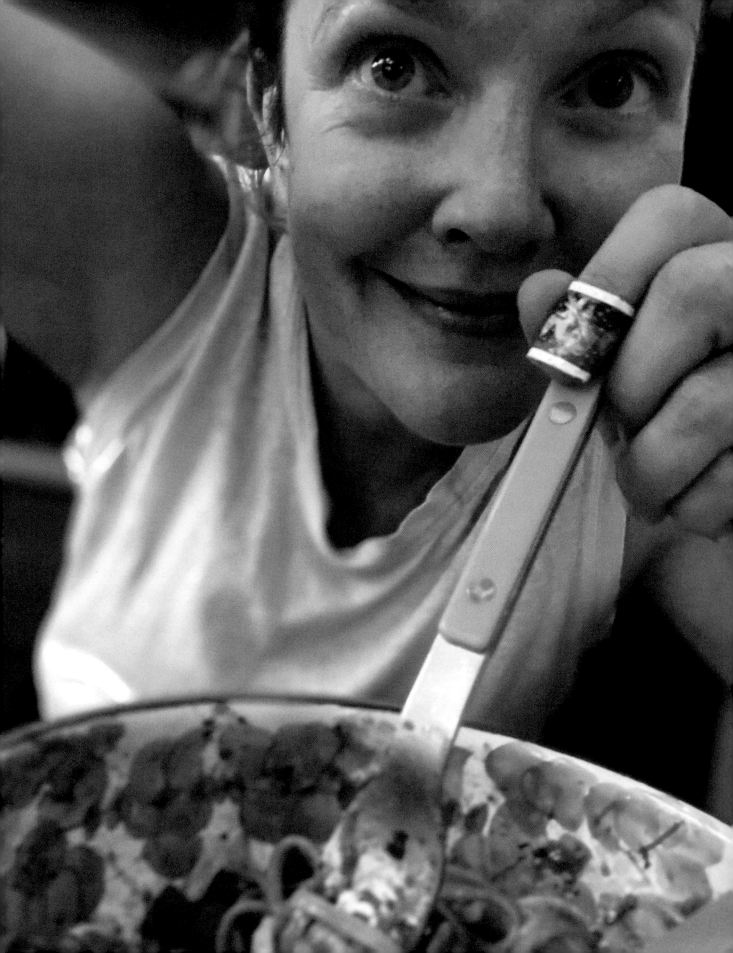

Who Am I to Write a Cookbook?

It's been two years—and two years I could have never predicted—since I decided to write a cookbook. In late 2019, I made a deal with my wonderful editor, Jill Schwartzman, with whom I did my last book, *Wildflower*, and I knew I was in trusted, safe, inspiring hands. And I knew that I would write it arm in arm with Pilar Valdes, my culinary partner in crime. I knew that the three of us, and some other integral people, would write a cookbook.

Wow, I would write a cookbook? I never thought that would ever happen. I think because way back in the 1990s, when I was at an impressionable age, all these life-style "gurus" seemed so perfect to me: "Follow me; do as I do." I know well that isn't me—I am messy and will be a student until the day I die. I am convinced that the right track in life is to be able to pivot to be a teacher if need be, but to still be that constantly curious researcher. How, how, how?

> **So something really did have to change, and it took me years to figure out exactly what those transitions were.**

I never thought I would have so much to do with food and design and making products. When I was a teenager the only thing I could see myself doing was making movies, so I started Flower Films at nineteen and spent the next fifteen years completely focused on that. We made a whole bunch of movies and had a whole lot of fun, although I probably stressed through it way more than I should have. Now, looking back, I see a young, invincible idiot who thought stress would never kill me and I would live forever. And now, at forty-six, I am going to try to take you on the journey of the two years just trying to make this book.

As of two years ago, I was in my midforties, I had two young daughters, and I was about to start a talk show. I'd spent the previous decade trying to pivot in my occupational aspirations so that I could keep all the research I have done in my life with me, and not negate my life's work. But I also knew that being a mom was my first priority now, and it would never be second to work again. So something really did have to change, and it took me years to figure out exactly what those transitions were. I decided to slow down on movies and started building brands. The very first one I created was Flower Beauty, a decade ago, and that company was born while I was birthing my two daughters. I was pregnant, with pigment swatches up and down my arms, as I got into the world and the marketing and the messaging of beauty.

Now this is an important detail, because looking back at my life and my youth in Hollywood, I knew somehow not to fall prey to vanity. I saw women around

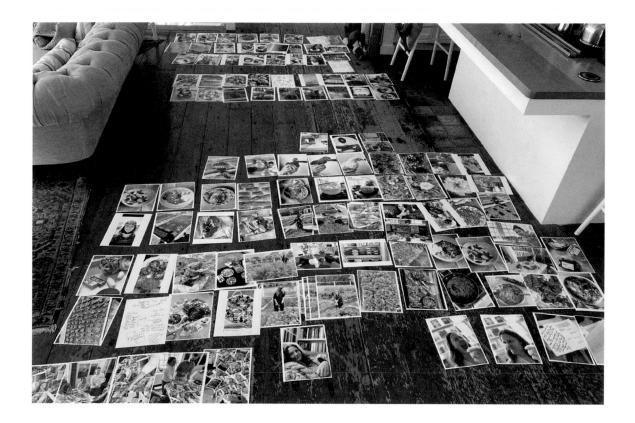

me looking rather tightly wound and worried about the way they looked and self-conscious about their bodies, and somehow, even as a little girl, I knew that did not look like a very easy way to live. However, I also noticed that when a woman walked into a dressing room to get her hair and makeup done, she'd come back out empowered. She'd look taller and more confident and that impression was really important to me.

And the question for me was born—what is beauty? Well, for me beauty is not about the way you look but about the way you feel. Beauty for me is something that you see outside of yourself, around you in the world. It's being able to recognize it and having the artistic ability to create it around yourself as well.

As a young girl who grew up around the world, working from job to job, location to location, I knew that I was lucky, because it made me very aware of the many different types of lives lived everywhere. It also gave me an extremely eclectic appetite for food and design. The more I traveled, the more I fell in love with everything I could get my eyes on and in my mouth. And finally, somewhere in my midtwenties, I became a true homemaker, realizing that traveling all the time was so tiring and expensive, and that I really did have no anchor in the world. So maybe the zip code 90046, a neighborhood I had lived in since I was born and never strayed from for long, maybe that was my home?

I'd found the place where I truly thought my roots would never be cut off. A house on Curson Terrace, right in the 90046; a house that I'd spend the next twenty years making a home, the anchor I had always wanted, with all the things I had collected throughout my life. My daughters were born, and I brought them through the threshold of that home thinking we would be there forever. I idealized it all—that my kids would have it different than I did. My kids would be able to come back to their childhood home when they were older, and they would be able to sleep in the rooms they were raised in.

But then guess what happened??? Life surprises you, and through marriage as well as divorce, I would find myself somehow on the island of Manhattan. I say that with an almost laughing-at-life luck because as a California girl, even though I traveled the world, I always battled Manhattan. The second I would land at any of the nearby airports, I felt like I was plugging into a human electrical socket. Manhattan, a place that I would associate with sleepless nights and partying. I lived in three neighborhoods—the East Village, the West Village, and the Upper West Side. I had lived many lives in Manhattan, and yet I never thought I would live there. All my stints were for months, a few years at most. They were fantasy, they were pretend role-play and make-believe all wrapped up in one burrito. (And as a California girl, I finally found one restaurant that actually has authentic California Mexican and I ordered from it, maybe too often), but never did I think Manhattan would claim me like it did during the winter of my divorce.

It was a hard time. Lightless, gray, wet, soggy days trying to find a rental apartment, wishing I could run back to California so badly, but I knew that would separate my daughters from the other half of their family, and I would do no such thing. I would remain in Manhattan so everybody could stay together. And I struggled for the next several years to try to figure out a way to make Manhattan a place I felt comfortable. The truth is I just kept running back to California, to the house I'd brought my daughters home to from the hospital. We would spend spring break, Christmas, and all summer in Los Angeles. I would pretend that we just went to school in New York and that we really lived in California, and as the years went by, having one foot in two places with three thousand miles between them, I realized I could not pull off this double life anymore.

I realized I would have to fully commit to being an East Coast girl. My kids were settled in school, and we were living right near their grandparents and their dad and their cousins. But I was living in a rental, and I knew that I had to make some type of final decision. It was one of the most difficult decisions I've ever made in my life. I sold the California house where I had thought we would grow up and maybe even grow old. Our lives have taken us east, another chapter of the book that makes up our beautiful lives. After years of pretending I could live in both places, it was over. One person saw the house on a pocket listing—it never hit the market—and the house was sold immediately.

I had ripped the Band-Aid off my life. Where was I going to go next? And how would I find a way to stay close to nature? Because I think that's what gets to me about Manhattan: the lack of green outdoor space. Don't get me wrong—I've learned to love it here. I guess I don't really have to prove it anymore, now that I live in Manhattan. I am a Manhattan girl now! I subscribe to *New York* magazine, and I call myself a proud New Yorker.

But I decided, after several years of living in Manhattan, that maybe we could

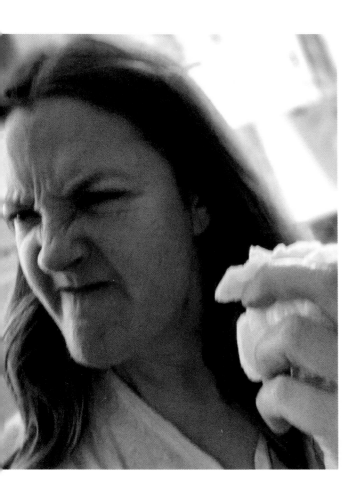

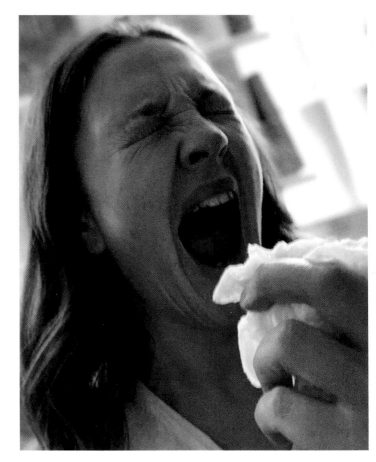

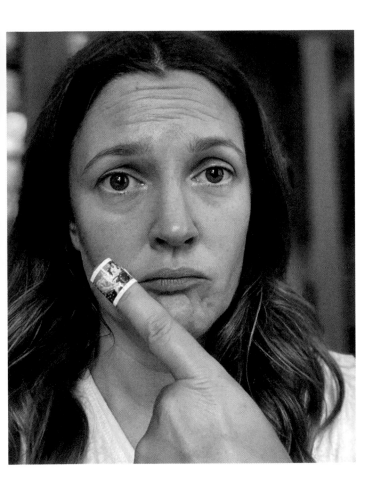
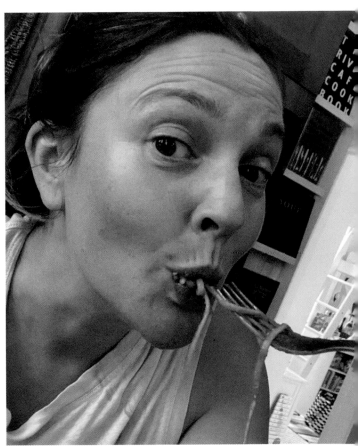

find a little place with a yard that has some trees, things that just get me back to my roots of who I am. How do I find my West Coast in the east? Well, I went looking, and I bought a house outside the city. Then six months later, the pandemic hit. And to my surprise, my daughters and I lived in it for the next eight months, without leaving. On the docket was virtual school for my two girls all day long, and then all afternoon I would fight to get the talk show I was developing off the ground—every day was lather, rinse, repeat.

I was all by myself with the girls for several months and I found capacities inside myself I didn't know I had, although, gosh, none of it looked pretty or felt good. I think I slowly unraveled, and yet I felt things I didn't know possible. The truth is when things are taken away, other things grow up in the now negative space. Human beings cannot be stopped—we are innovative creatures; we find a way.

And eventually we found a new groove. Despite how strange things were, with businesses closed and schools remote, and despite a level of fear unlike anything anyone had experienced before, I did my best. As we lived there over the next eight months, I tried to set up the house as best as I was able, unpacking our California moving boxes and organizing everything I could. But there wasn't much energy left after school and trying to get the show off the ground. I would help my girls with Zoom school from 8:00 a.m. till 2:00 p.m., and then from 2:00 p.m. till 7:00 p.m. I would be on Zooms trying to launch my talk show. At the end of each day I was maxed out. But I wanted to help my girls focus on something that represented life when we were so afraid of death itself, so I thought, what else can I do right now?

So for the first time in my life, I bought some chickens. My daughters and I went to a hatchery to get six tiny chicks. We brought them home and put them under a heat lamp so they could grow big and strong. Looking back, I realize how much I turn to nature when faced with the peril of mortality. I also decided I would plant my very first vegetable garden. Again, I don't want to sound like some '90s life-

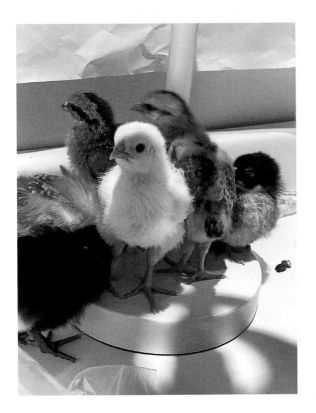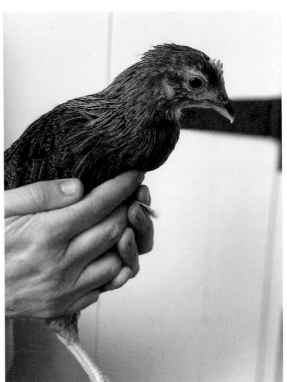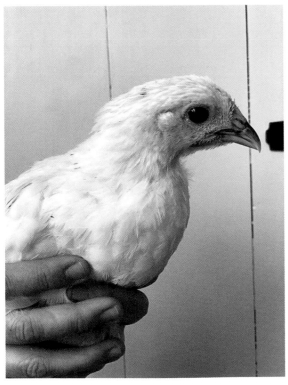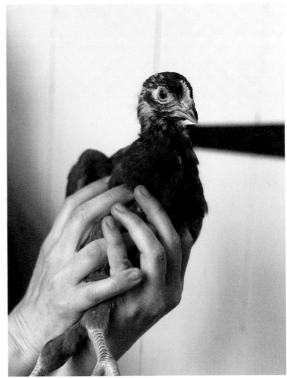

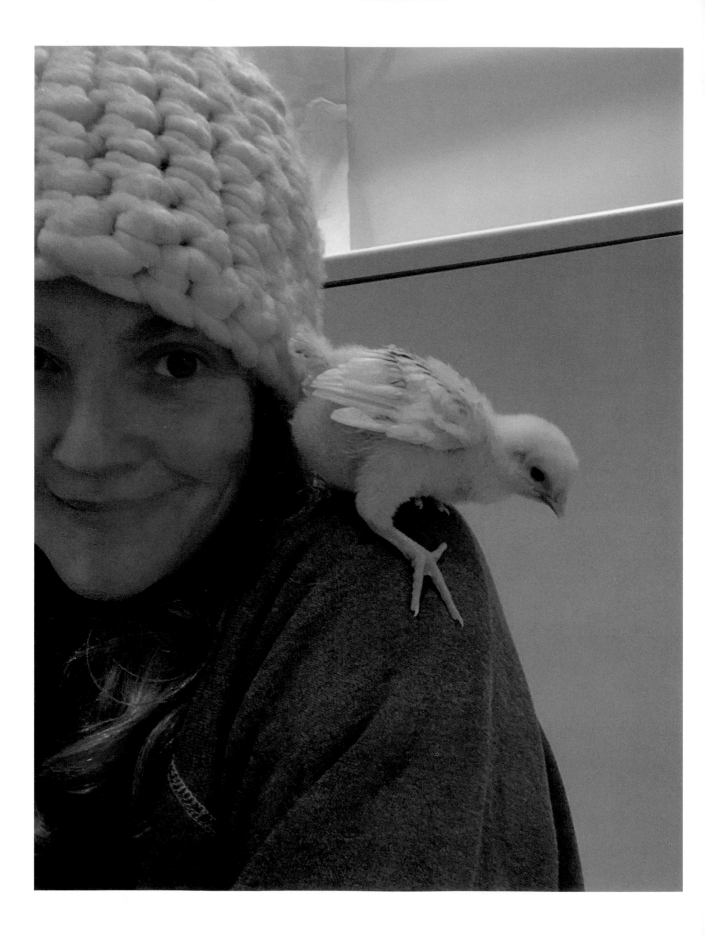

style guru. Please don't roll your eyes and think, "Oh, you eat your own produce that you grow in your garden? Wow, you're so amazing." I'll *never* be that person.

And with life still feeling like it was hanging in the balance and all of us locked inside, I took my yard, which was completely bare when I bought the house—it was really just a wonderful blank canvas of brown grass—and went to work. I learned how to plant vegetable boxes so we could eat the food I grew. I started becoming my own landscaper, taking trips to the nursery and buying trees for the property. I learned what perennials and evergreens are. I learned which plants bloom when and what their Latin names are. I really decided to throw myself wholeheartedly into this project. Working alongside nature and watching from March until June was so inspiring, because it literally went from brown grass right into beautiful blooming floral life.

The chickens grew and started to look really different, and finally moved outside from under the heat lamp.

The chickens grew and started to look really different, and finally moved outside from under the heat lamp. We wish they had laid eggs, but they weren't old enough yet. Still, this little blank canvas started to take beautiful shape and truly come alive. By the end of the summer of 2020, I was back in Manhattan and somehow we had gotten our little show off the ground.

Now it was September, and we were in a studio, carefully filming preshows with strict regulations, and rehearsing and polishing and getting ready for our big debut.

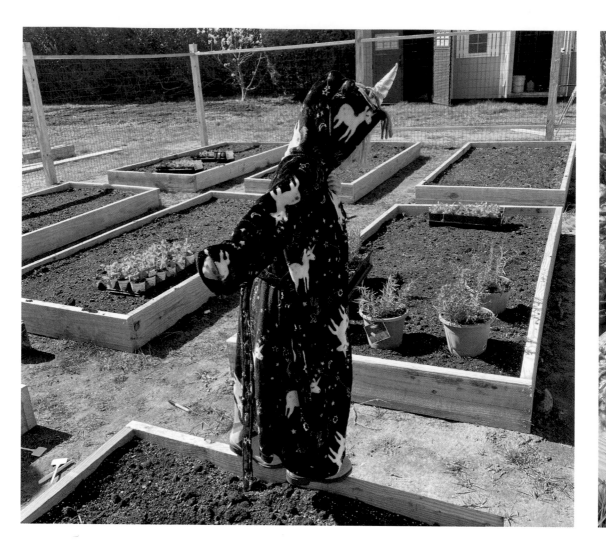

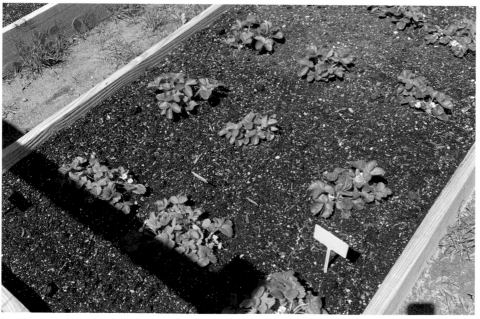

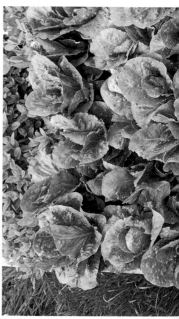

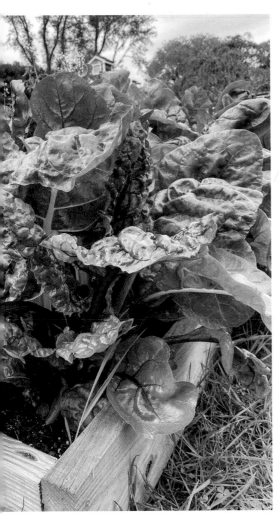

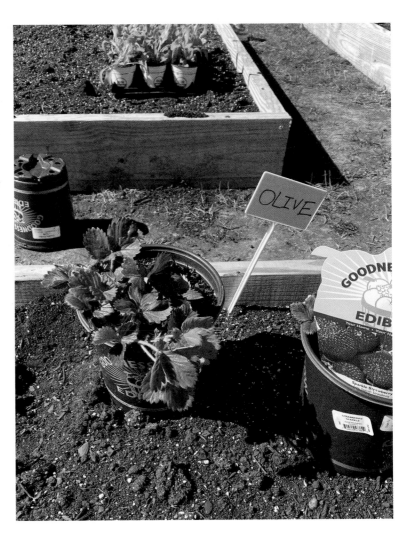

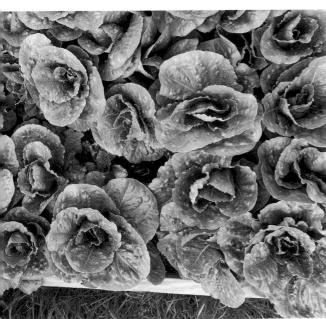

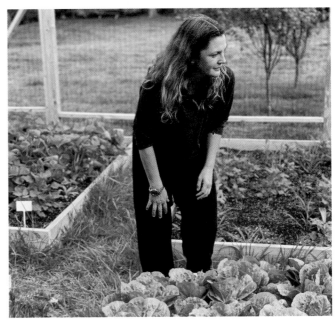

In a studio with no audience, in the middle of an insane political crisis, in the middle of a changing Supreme Court, in the middle of an election, in the middle of the Black Lives Matter movement, in the middle of the global pandemic. How could someone squeak through all that and come on TV and not look totally nutty? I felt nutty, but true to form, I threw myself entirely into it: I hired a teacher because I would no longer be able to do the homeschool by myself, and I started my new job.

As I write this, it is now the following spring. We are one year after the pandemic hit, and I am writing stories for this book. I did a lot of writing during the pandemic as well—again, when so many other things shut down, you find new things—so I started a blog and told Jill, my editor, that writing was not eluding me, even in the midst of all this craziness. That we were going to make this book very personal and eclectic and messy and real, and that no matter what, no matter how hard we worked on the book, it couldn't be too polished. I don't want to be the late '90s lifestyle guru that I could never relate to. I don't wanna be a fraud; I wanna be utterly myself—how can I put me into this book?

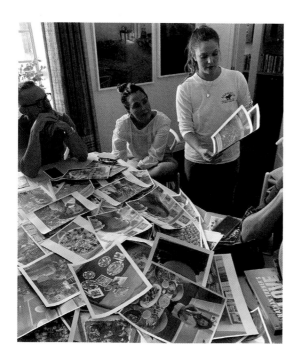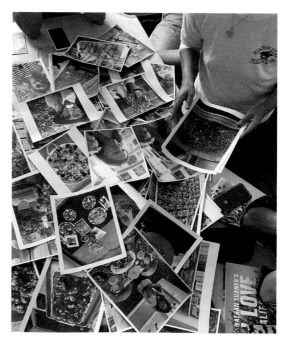

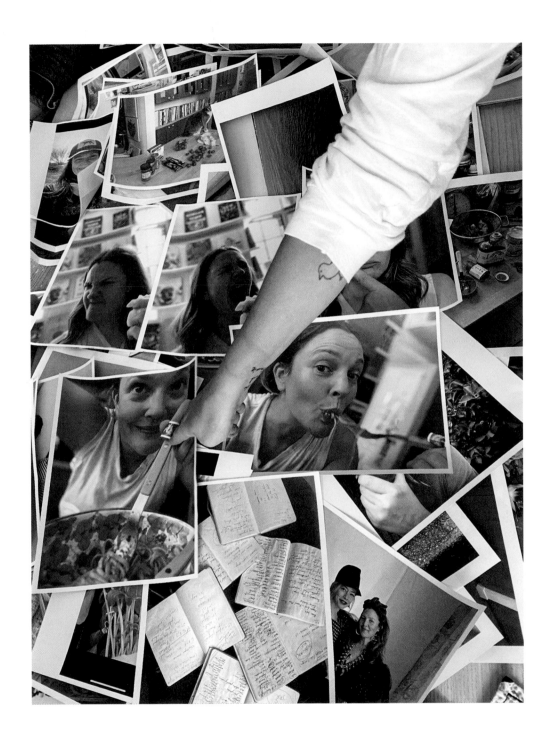

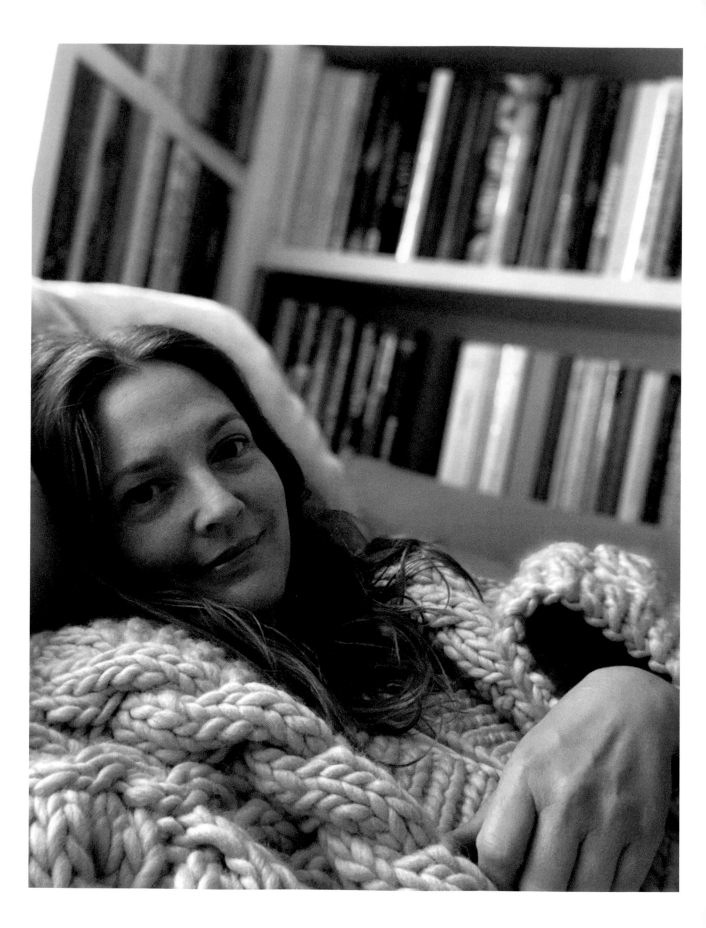

Well, one way was that I started printing out photos of my real life instead of having every image taken by a professional photographer in a studio and then airbrushed. I knew this book could be different if I put my own photography into it. But later, after living with just my photos for months, I realized, you know what? Some professional shots of the food might be nice, and we found the best photographers, the Graydon/Herriott team. I needed some level of aspiration—not just reality—so we found a really nice happy medium, and then I wrote all the stories for the book.

If I can't have a sense of humor about it, I won't make it in this world.

Pilar Valdes, who I've been cooking with for years, and I worked tirelessly on all the recipes, adding and editing each and every ingredient. Pilar worked with an incredible recipe developer named Nora Singley. I set them up for success by saying, "Look at this commercial where the girl is trying to cook dinner for her date and her dad is telling her how to go through it. Guess what, since none of us are allowed to be together, you guys are going to be that commercial." I set them up on FaceTime, and they started writing and concocting. Pilar and I were in a bubble, so we would cook and taste everything, and then Pilar and Nora would write the actual recipes. I would take my own photographs of our cooking sessions, and eventually, we got to take it prime time to the professionals and have a bunch of our dishes photographed as well.

It's been a long time coming, this book, and since the fall of 2019, much life will have been lived. And I'm hoping that this book can be a reflection of all of that, and of what I've learned. And probably the most important thing I've come to realize is that as much as I was always looking for an anchor in the form of a home, I've fallen

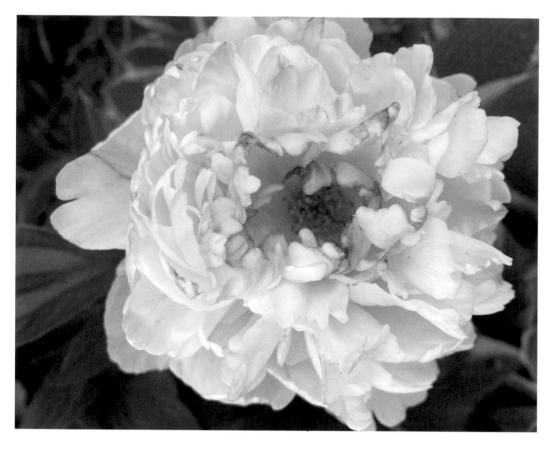

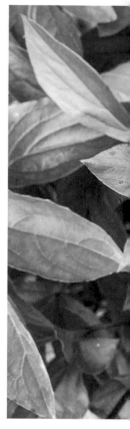

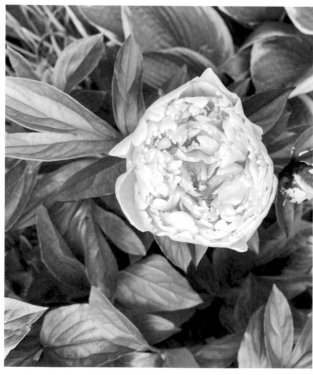

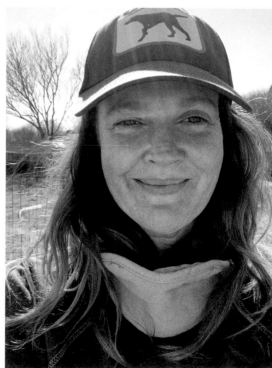

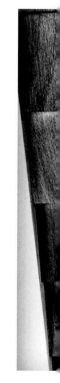

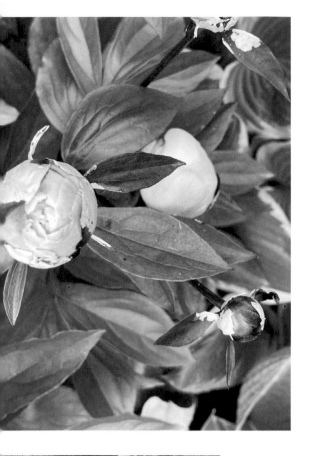

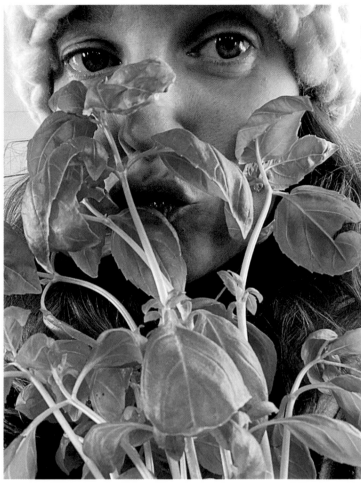

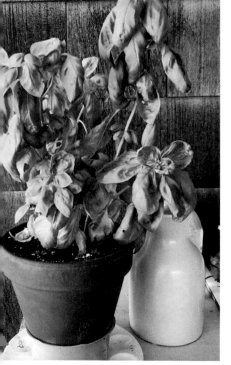

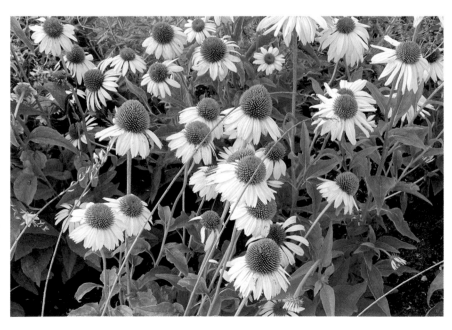

I realized I am a Rebel Homemaker through and through.

in love with the saying "Home is where the heart is," because anywhere my girls and I are together, we will find happiness.

And that realization, and our current version of home, is probably exactly where we are supposed to be. I no longer have the notion of what it's all supposed to look like, and how home should function a certain way. All my original plans got blown up, and if I can't have a sense of humor about it, I won't make it in this world. Life continues to show me that you have to be malleable and adaptable and able to pivot. That's the kind of resilience I am talking about. Personally, I'm not very good at being idle. We have to put one foot in front of the other and keep going.

Within the two years that I've spent making this book, I will have fully departed from California, truly become an East Coaster, started a talk show, survived a year of homeschool, written a cookbook, and did half the photography for it! Then, as I wrote the essays, I realized I had to explain what I think a homemaker is. When Jill and I discussed ideas for the title, nothing was really landing. We were in the middle of a global crisis and everything felt too prissy or too trite or too hoity-toity. And one day during one of our conversations, as we banged our heads against the wall trying to shape this book over Zoom, I came up with *Rebel Homemaker*. The reason I love the word "rebel" is because it's totally bombastic without being angry—it's someone who's just like me. I can't stand rules, and even when I try to create them, they blow up in my face. We need structure, we need social agreements, but we also need societal openheartedness and progressive ways to take care of one another.

I realized I am a Rebel Homemaker through and through. I grew up in an unorthodox way where I spent my whole life around the entire globe, and then finally settled down in my twenties, bought a house, and thought I'd live there forever, as

I've said. But the truth is that it was two incredible decades, and it was a chapter in my larger story. Life goes on, home is where we are, and if we are not adaptive and able to pivot, well, 2020 really showed us. None of us have any choice, and we have to rise to whatever occasions are thrown at us.

But how can I take my whole life experience of traveling and loving food and wanting to be a homemaker and put it all in a book? By the way, side note, when I looked up the historic definition of "homemaker" I got even more rebellious—for generations, it was assumed that the woman was the homemaker, and therefore it meant she stayed in the home. There was a societal agreement that she was not the breadwinner or even had any purpose outside the home. In my humble opinion, we need to update the definition to be as modern as our current world. It's time to strip away the layers of conformity surrounding words and titles and redefine the ones we as individuals don't feel represent us.

I am a passionate homemaker, but I've also been a lifelong worker bee, so how can I modernize the term "homemaker" as well as throw a "rebel" in it? Because I'm a woman taking care of my home and my children, and I'm the breadwinner, and I do so much more than that, and I don't wanna be stopped! I want to be able to do well in business as well as grow a garden and raise chickens. I want to be a mother first and someone who knows and lives by the fact that my kids come first. Well, creating that balance between work and home was definitely an amazing, if forced, experiment during these past two years.

I am also a messy home cook. I spill, I splatter, and I laugh. I run around not prepping things properly and portioning things out. Pilar is so much smarter and better at all these things, and she has made me such a better cook. She's made it so much less stressful and so much more fun for me. Maybe we all need partners, one way or another? I haven't done anything by myself—Flower Films, Flower Beauty, Flower anything. My talk show doesn't exist solely because of me; nothing in this world really does. I think I come alive when I find a partner. This also makes me shun the "lifestyle guru" label because my biggest thing is to shine a light on the people who are showing me how to do it, not me teaching people how to do it. Again, I go back to the fact that I am a student, and I will forever be a student, humble, excited, and passionate.

I also love being a curator. That's what I do on the show, and that's what I do in this book. I have discovered and found all these wonderful things. Let me share them with you. Share, not show. Show gives an air of arrogance.

So let me share my life with you. Let me share this book with you. Let me share my journey. Let me share the new experiences I've had these two years, like growing a garden and raising chickens. By the way, they finally started laying their eggs! And now I am an official egg snob—I only want *their* eggs.

I love creating my own opportunities. Whether it be a national talk show or my very first tiny vegetable garden and everything in between, I am a curator and a creator. We all are! We are cultivators, and if we ever get scared and lost, we should turn to nature so that it can show us that things have cycles. And if cycles exist, then chapters exist. Our narratives are ever changing, and you must bring everything you've experienced with you. You have to fight and choose to be happy where you are now.

I never knew at age forty-six I would be a New Yorker, with two daughters and a full-time diversified job that I am so proud of, where I get to talk about food and design, and share my love of life and of relationships. And human stories, celebrating the incredible things happening all around us. The pandemic brought empathy and humanity and taking care of each other to the forefront. So let's celebrate human capacity—the greatest challenges and the smallest wins and everything in between. And let's find out if we are lucky enough to be homemakers with no definition to box us in and define us, and then let's celebrate life and finding your own rebel homemaker and share what we've all learned along the way.

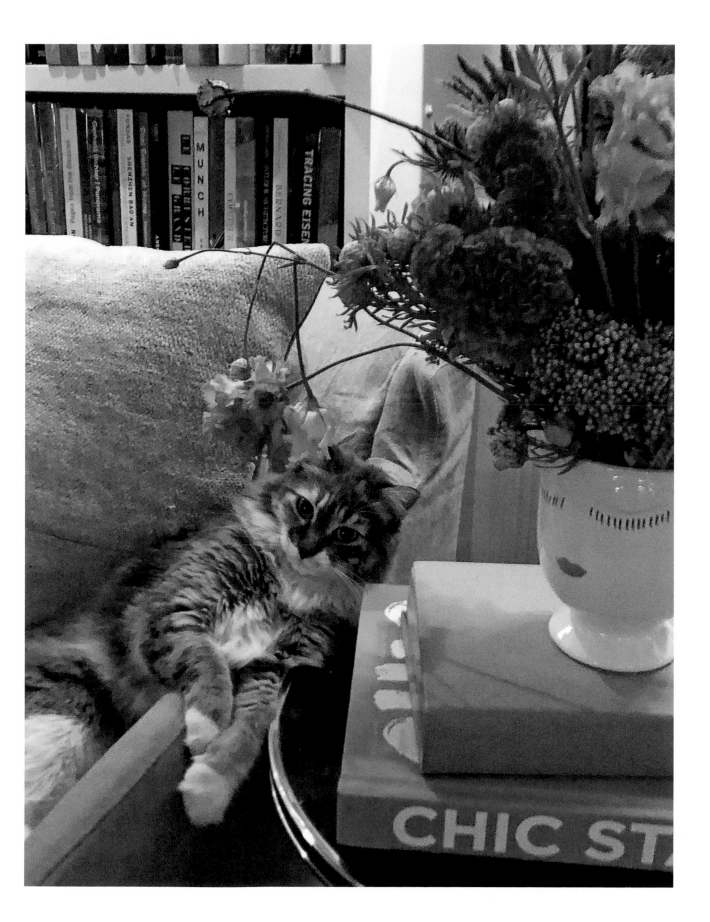

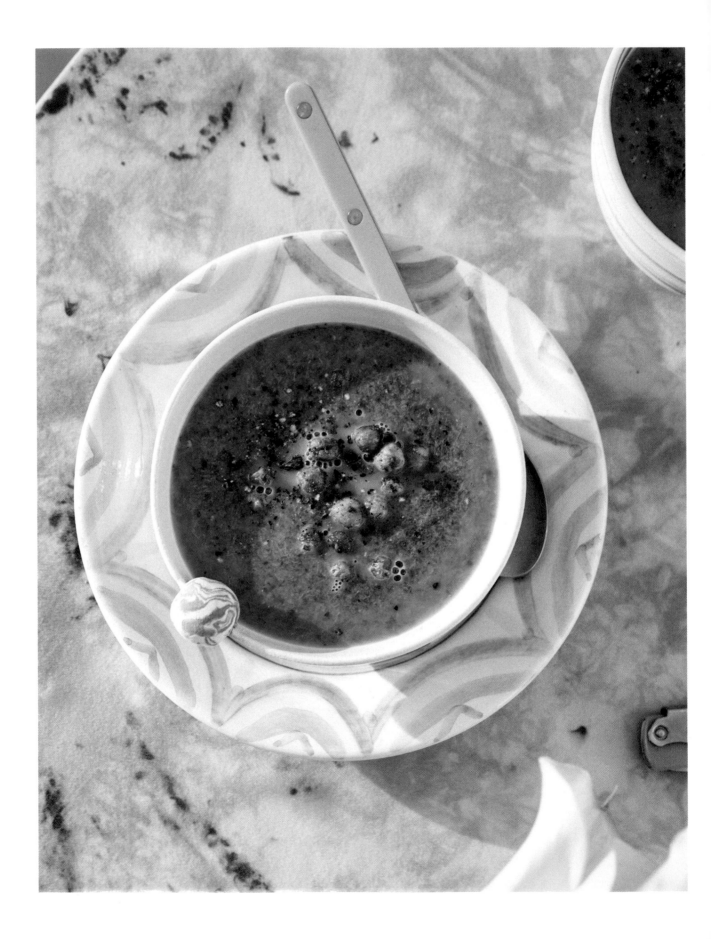

1 (15.5-ounce) can garbanzo
  beans, drained and
  rinsed; aquafaba (bean-
  soaking liquid) reserved

2 tablespoons plus
  2 teaspoons olive oil,
  divided

1 teaspoon ground sumac

Kosher salt and freshly
  ground black pepper

½ teaspoon coriander seed

2 cups sliced leeks, about
  2 small leeks (white and
  light green parts only)

2½ cups water, plus
  additional as necessary

1 (6-ounce) bunch flat-leaf
  spinach, stems included,
  roughly chopped

1 (4-ounce) bunch watercress,
  stems included, roughly
  chopped

Flaky sea salt (we love
  Maldon), for serving
  (optional)

All the Greens:
Spinach-Watercress Soup

Soup for breakfast! This recipe is incredibly simple and really delicious—and it just so happens to be vegan and jam-packed with a ton of dark greens. We love the combination of watercress for its peppery bite and super health benefits, and flat-leaf, vitamin-packed spinach, but feel free to experiment with other greens like kale, swiss chard, or even dandelion greens.

The crispy garbanzo garnish can be made 5 days in advance (and it also makes a great healthy snack). The rest of the recipe takes about 15 minutes to make, which keeps things nice and simple. Easy like Sunday morning.

Make the crispy garbanzos. Preheat the oven to 475 degrees. Measure out ½ cup of the garbanzo beans and set aside. Place the remaining garbanzo beans on a small rimmed baking sheet and pat dry with a paper towel. Drizzle with 2 teaspoons olive oil and shake the baking sheet to coat. Season with sumac, and salt and pepper. Shake the baking sheet again to distribute the spices evenly. Transfer to the oven and roast until the garbanzos are crispy and golden on the edges, 20 to 25 minutes, stirring halfway through. Reserve for serving. (Crispy garbanzos can be made up to 5 days in advance, stored in an airtight container at room temperature.)

Make the soup. Meanwhile, heat a large pot over medium-high heat. Add the remaining 2 tablespoons of olive oil, swirl to coat, and add the coriander seeds and leeks. Season with salt and pepper and sauté, stirring occasionally, until softened and just beginning to brown, 4 to 5 minutes, reducing the heat as necessary to prevent burning.

Add the aquafaba, reserved ½ cup garbanzo beans, and water. Raise the heat to high and bring to a boil. Add the spinach and watercress to the pot and return to a boil. Cook, stirring, until the greens are wilted, about 1 minute.

Transfer mixture to a blender and blend until the soup is very smooth, adding additional water 1 tablespoon at a time if necessary to thin to your desired consistency. Season to taste with additional salt and pepper.

Serve. Ladle soup into 4 bowls and top with the crispy garbanzos, freshly cracked black pepper, and flaky sea salt. (The soup should have a brothy consistency. Since we are not straining it, some separation may occur—just stir until fully combined before serving.)

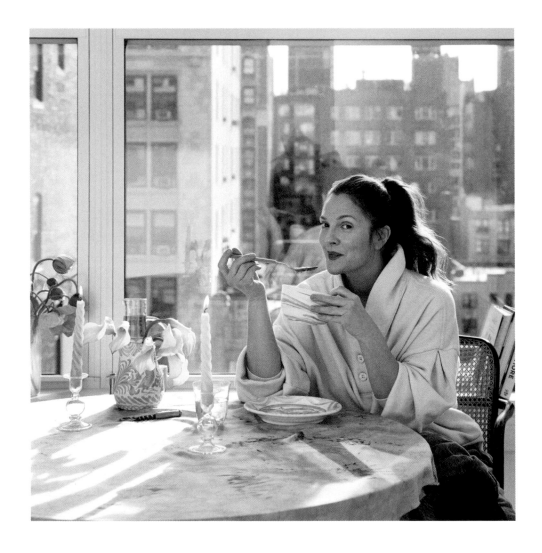

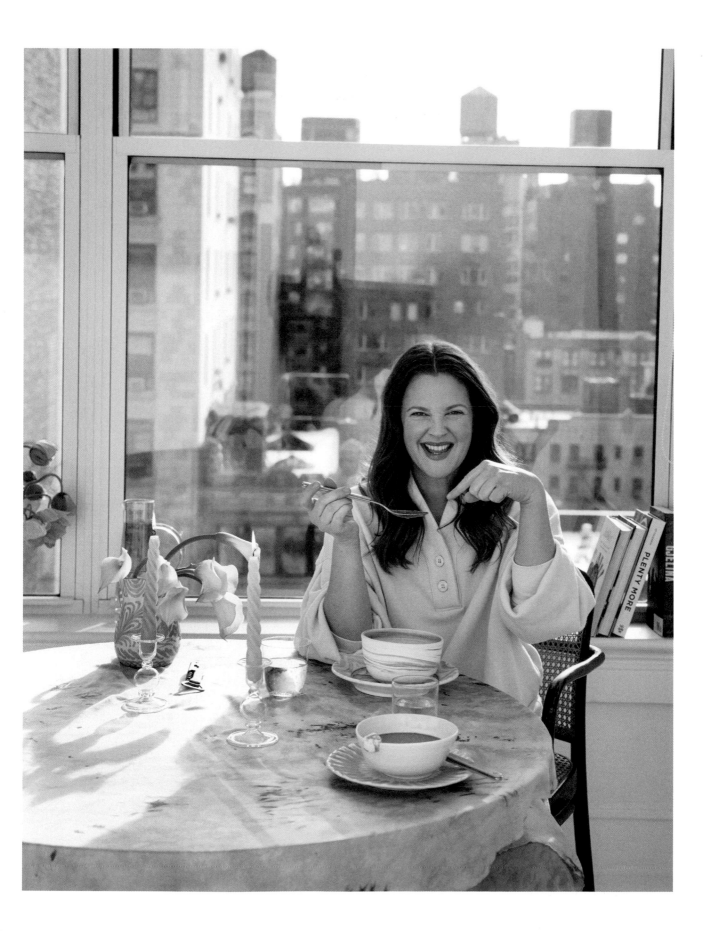

Sunrise Quinoa Porridge

MAKES 5 CUPS
SERVES 4

*For Homemade
Vegetable Stock*
(To Make 7 Cups)

2 tablespoons olive oil

**3 large shallots, peeled and
roughly chopped (¾ cup)**

**2 cloves garlic, peeled and
smashed**

**1 leek, roughly chopped, about
2 heaping cups (white and
light green parts only)**

**Kosher salt and freshly
ground black pepper**

**1 large beefsteak tomato,
roughly chopped (about
2 cups)**

**2 stalks celery, plus leaves,
cut into 3-inch pieces**

**6 ounces cremini mushrooms,
sliced (about 2 cups)**

½ bunch parsley

4 sprigs thyme

3 dried bay leaves

10 cups water

(ingredients continue)

Yet another soup for breakfast! Asian porridges made from rice (sometimes known as congee) are often enjoyed in the morning. It's a culinary practice embraced all around the world, and I absolutely adore it.

I loooove rice, but sometimes I have to cut back on eating (too much of) it, so Pilar came up with this comforting quinoa porridge. Pureeing part of the soup base helps give it a thicker, satisfying consistency—which is a nod to our love of congee.

We've included the recipe of our Homemade Vegetable Stock (which can be made ahead and frozen for up to 3 months), but feel free to substitute a store-bought vegetable stock or even just plain water.

I love having this soup for breakfast on early shoot days because it's so comforting and gives me protein and energy. We finish the dish with herbs for those beautiful pops of freshness and flavor.

Make the stock. Heat a large pot over medium-high heat. Add the olive oil and swirl to coat. Add the shallots, garlic, and leek. Season with salt and pepper and sauté, stirring, until the vegetables are softened and translucent, 5 to 6 minutes. Reduce heat, if necessary, to prevent browning. Add the tomato, celery, mushrooms, parsley, thyme, bay leaves, water, and 2 teaspoons of salt. Bring to a boil and continue to cook until the liquid is reduced by about a quarter, 20 to 25 minutes. Remove from heat, strain through a fine-mesh strainer, and discard the solids. You should have 7 cups of stock. Keep in mind that liquid reduces at different rates on every stovetop, so you may need to add a touch of water or continue reducing to make 7 cups. (The stock can be made in advance. Keep in the refrigerator, covered in an airtight container, up to 3 days, or in the freezer for up to 3 months.)

Make the soup. Place a medium pot over medium heat. Add the quinoa and toast, stirring frequently, until the quinoa is fragrant and a hue darker, about 2 minutes. Remove the pot from the heat and very slowly pour in the stock, being very careful as it will

For the Quinoa

1 cup white quinoa

7 cups vegetable stock (homemade or store bought)

1 tablespoon chopped fresh dill, divided

Zest of 1 lemon

1 scallion, thinly sliced

spatter. Return to the heat, adjust to maintain a brisk simmer, and cook, stirring occasionally, until the quinoa is fully cooked and starts to break down, 12 to 14 minutes. Season to taste with salt.

Transfer half of the mixture to a blender. Blend until smooth and return to the pot with the remaining cooked quinoa and heat through. Remove from the heat and stir in ½ tablespoon of dill. Check for seasoning. (As the quinoa soup sits, it will become thicker; thin to desired consistency if necessary, adding 1 tablespoon of water at a time.)

Serve. Ladle soup into bowls. Top with lemon zest, remaining dill, and sliced scallion.

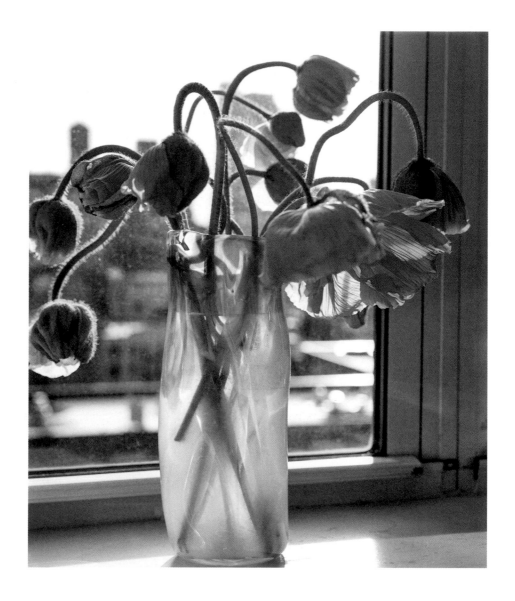

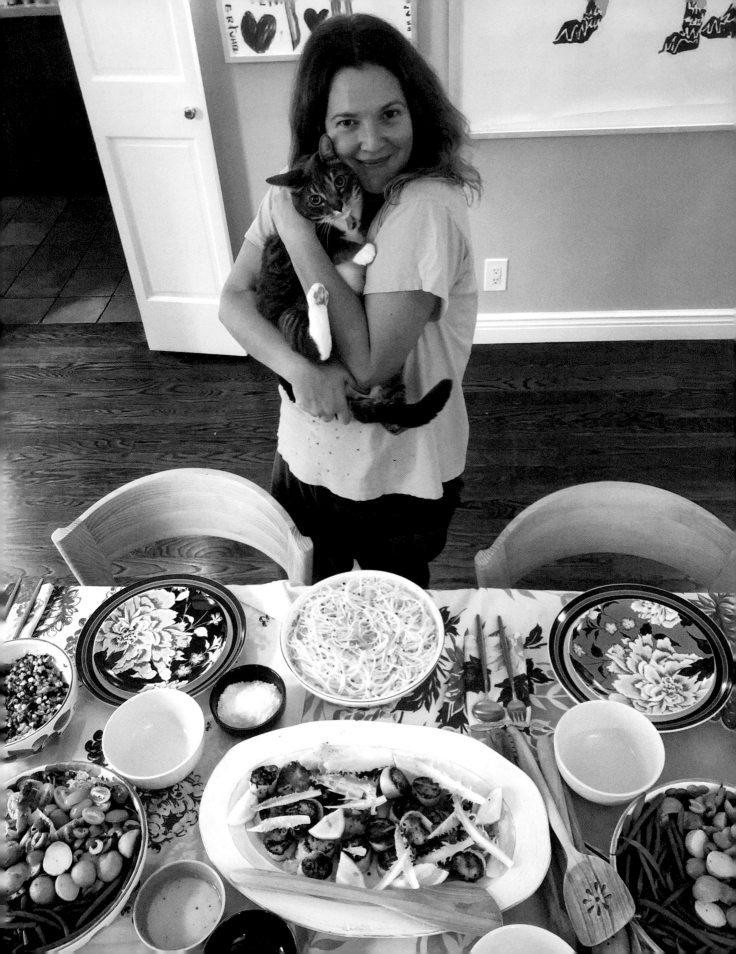

Creating a Space Where You Love to Cook and Eat

Drew: I'm an entertainer type. I really focus on tablescaping. Even before I knew it was called tablescaping, I was a big tablescaper. I always think about the greenery on the table or create a dried flower motif. Always very lo-fi, more wildflowers, not overly ornate, expensive florals. I don't find that necessary. I'd rather find unique little vases, layering in vintage floral tablecloths. I don't care if the plates are mixed—I just like to have something cohesive, like the tablecloth, and then I play from there. Mismatched napkins, or you can keep it neutral or colorful. I think setting the table is my favorite part. I always go interior designer on it!

Pilar: You always create welcoming and warm places. It always feels nice and special, and not fussy. People really appreciate that, and you have such a definitive stamp and style.

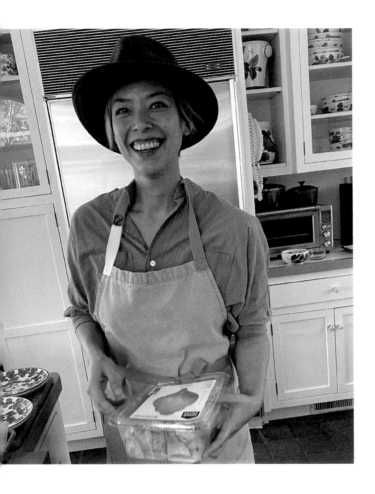

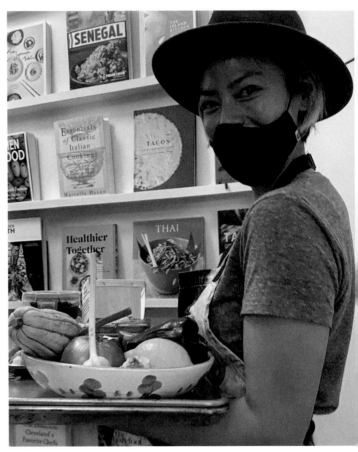

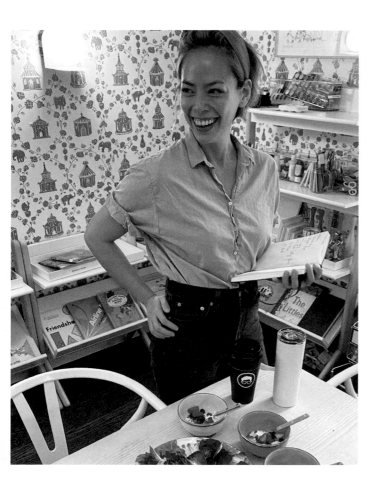

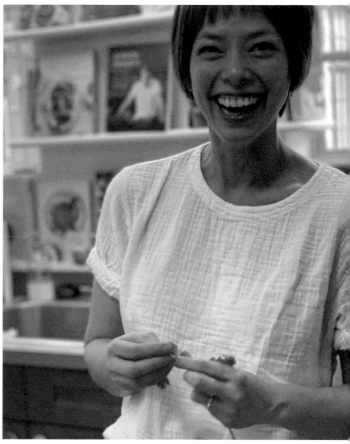

Drew: The last thing I want it to feel like is a wedding. I feel like some dinner parties are very place-settingy and formal, and that makes me uncomfortable. I want it to feel fluid. I want people to be at ease. I want the materials to be relaxed. I want the people to be relaxed.

Pilar: There's a certain level of looseness that you're able to create at your table. No matter how small or how large the gathering is, there's always a really warm feeling to it.

Drew: I love that we've started having everyone help themselves—and I think this is important because it's a table setting and the way you eat. It's unfussy to do big platters, shared plates, and served family style. Put it all on a table that everyone can serve from. Not buffet style, but put the plates on the big table itself. Whichever way you want to roll, keep it really loose.

Pilar: It has that energy. It's very convivial and very warm. I think people are so much more excited to be at a table where you can do that instead of thinking, "This fork or that fork?" That feels very uncomfortable.

Drew: I want to feel like I can get up from the table and that's acceptable. I want to take the formality out of it.

Here's a tip I really care about in tablescaping—too big of a round circle or too wide of a farm-style table will keep you too far removed from your dinner guests, and the conversation gets narrowed to about three people instead of five or six. A narrow farm table keeps everybody closer together. And don't make a round table too wide—if you have to, you should just shove everyone in and have a smaller one. Don't space people out too much, because you immediately lose more people to talk to, and you can only be in one or two conversations. It's not as communal. Put the communal in the communal table!

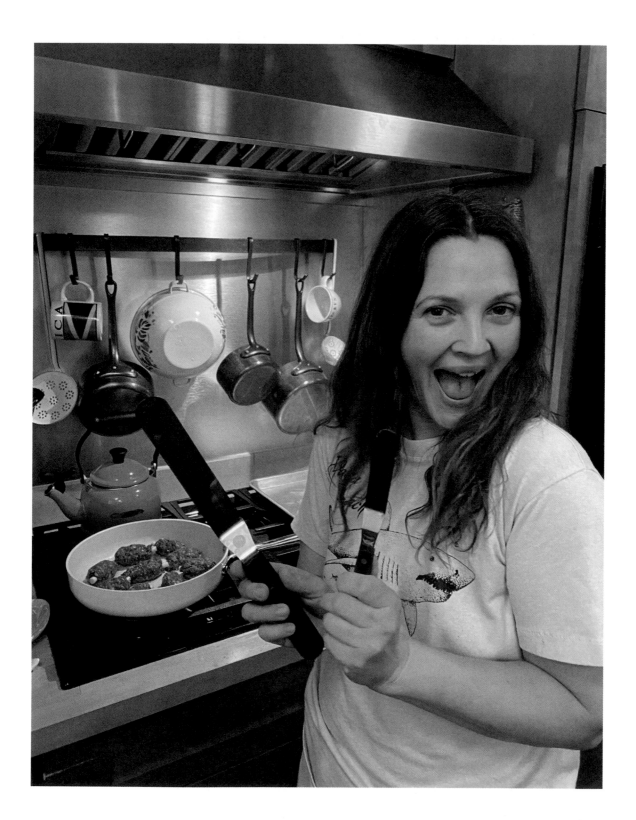

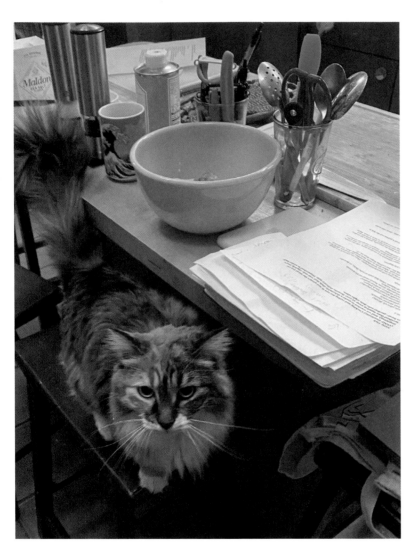

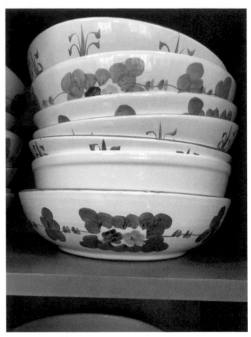

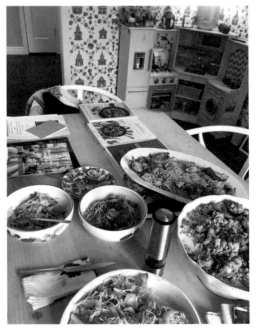

Pilar: As to the cooking aspect of that, we try to keep our menus really simple and accessible, and thoughtfully prepared. Unfussy, same as the table. So people feel good about what they're eating and what they're reaching for. When you cook, you want to make people happy. What do people love? What are they allergic to? So we can bring those pieces into the menu.

Drew: I also use that old food pyramid we were taught as children—a protein, a starch, a vegetable, a salad, a soup. But I want to diversify the types of food, and I am cajoling everyone to start traveling the world through food. I get really greedy in our meals—how many places can we travel? My friend Dina calls me EPCOT.

Pilar: We're going to visit Japan with this dish! And then Italy! When you create the menu, Drew, it's always a curation of your favorites, how you want to share that with people. And I always really, really appreciate that.

Drew: I think there's also a way to match flavors, so even if you're into different geographies of food origins, there's something that can bring them together. What are the spices and flavors that speak to each other so it feels more cohesive?

Pilar: Because you've traveled so much and eaten across the globe, you're really good at seeing that, and putting things together in a really interesting but unexpected way. I think, "Hmm, I never would have thought of that, but it works!" Sometimes it sounds bananas, but . . .

Drew: If there's one thing I know about me, it's that I'm bananas!

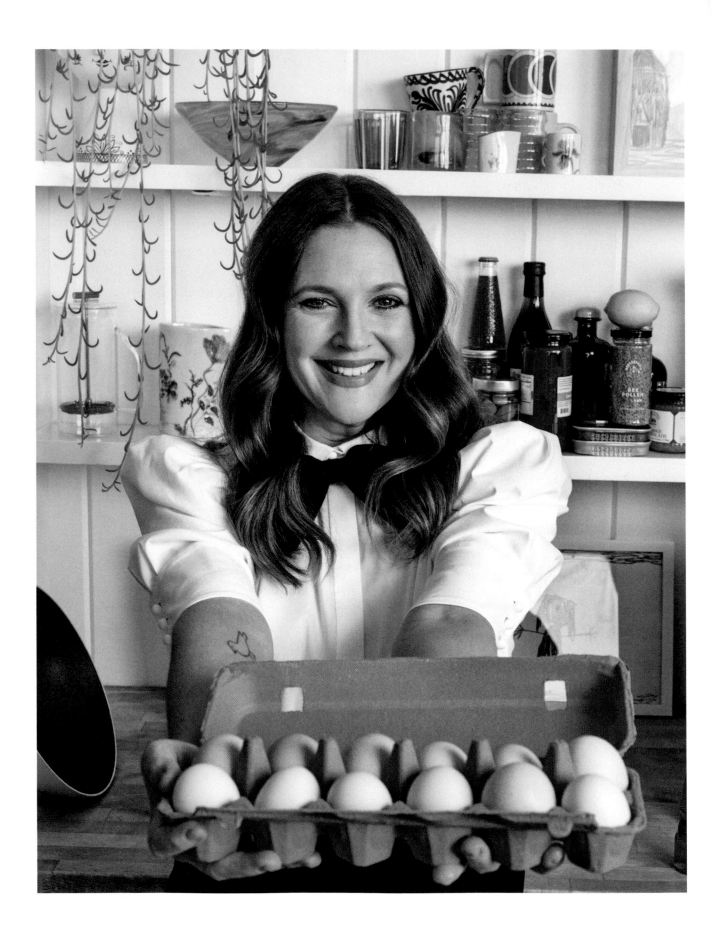

Dina's Breakfast Tacos

MAKES 8 TACOS

SERVES 4

1 tablespoon plus 2 teaspoons
olive oil, divided

1 green bell pepper, halved,
seeded, and cut lengthwise
into ½-inch strips

1 medium yellow onion, peeled
and cut lengthwise into
½-inch slices

Kosher salt and freshly
ground black pepper

2 teaspoons ground cumin

2 teaspoons sweet paprika

1 tablespoon freshly squeezed
lime juice, plus 2 limes cut
into wedges for serving

⅓ cup cilantro leaves and
stems, roughly chopped,
plus additional sprigs for
garnish

10 large eggs

8 small flour or corn tortillas

½ head iceberg lettuce,
roughly chopped

1 avocado, peeled, pitted,
and thinly sliced

Dina is one of my very favorite chefs. We met through a mutual friend and now I am an absolute devotee of her cooking. I asked her if she would give us a recipe for this book, so please meet one of the very best ways to start your day–or even end it, for that matter! "Eggs for Dinner" is never a bad idea.

The key to this dish is how she cooks the peppers and onions down with a smoked paprika. She tosses them in a pan until they are a perfect texture; and when I make it, I throw the peppers and onions in with the scrambled eggs into a tortilla topped with avocado, lettuce, and salsa. But I'm telling you, it's all about the peppers. And truth be told, this is simply one of my very favorite breakfasts on planet Earth.

Cook the bell peppers. Heat a large skillet over medium-high heat. Add 1 tablespoon olive oil and swirl to coat. Add the bell peppers and the onions, season with salt and pepper, and sauté, stirring, until just tender, about 4 minutes. Add the cumin and paprika and continue to cook until the spices are fragrant and toasted, about

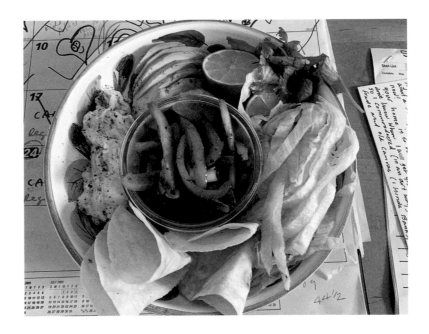

1 minute more. Transfer to a bowl and cover to keep warm. Just before serving, season with lime juice and salt to taste, and fold in the cilantro.

Wipe the skillet clean with a paper towel.

Make the eggs. Whisk the eggs in a large bowl. Season them with salt and pepper. Warm a large nonstick skillet over medium heat and add the remaining 2 teaspoons of olive oil and swirl to coat. Add the beaten eggs to the skillet. With a silicone spatula or wooden spoon, begin to stir, gently and continuously. Remove the skillet from the stovetop just before you reach the desired doneness, as the eggs will continue to cook off the heat.

Heat the tortillas. Using the same skillet you used for the bell peppers, heat over medium-high heat. Add one tortilla at a time, flipping to warm evenly, until the tortilla becomes soft and pliable (about 30 seconds). Wrap it in a dish towel to keep warm, and continue with the remaining tortillas.

Serve. Squeeze a few lime wedges over the avocado slices and season with salt. Divide tortillas among plates and top each one with a spoonful of sautéed onions and bell peppers, eggs, lettuce, and avocado slices. Serve immediately, garnished with additional cilantro, a wedge or two of lime, and salt and pepper on the side.

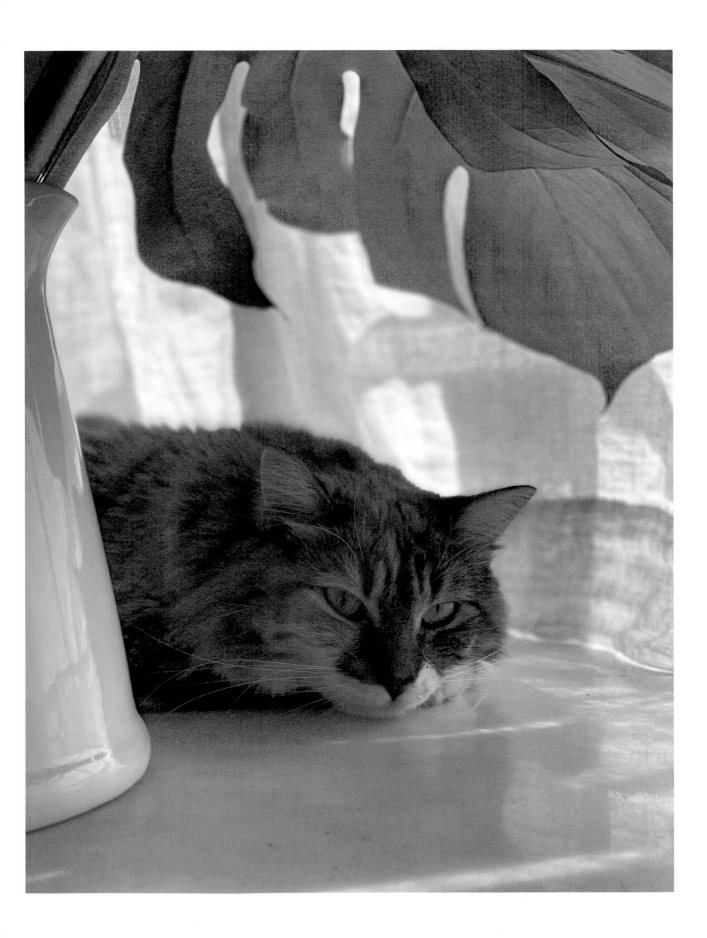

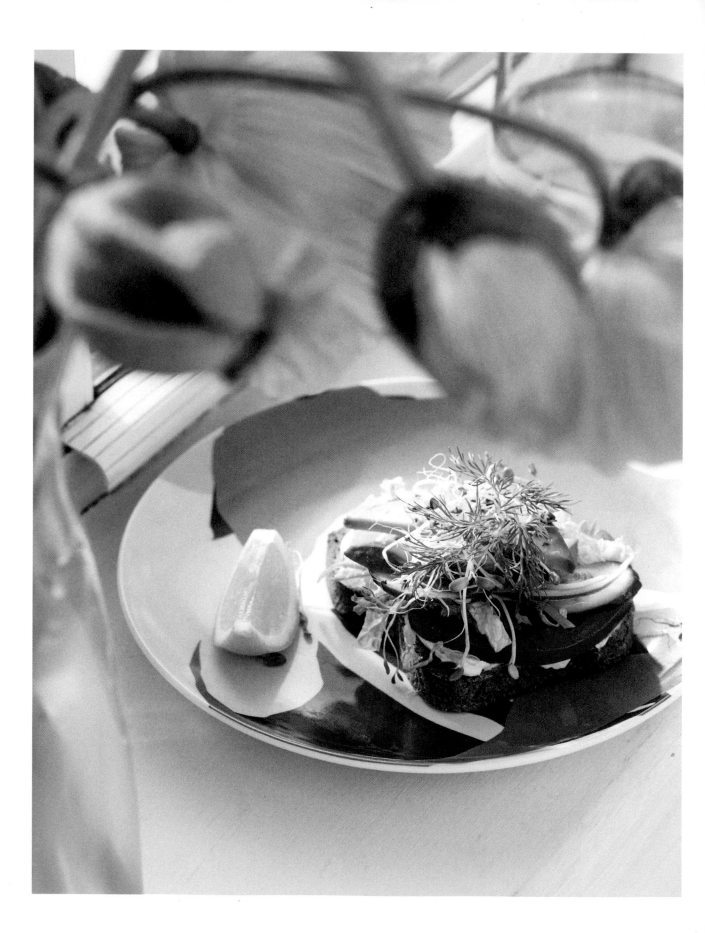

Drew's Cali Tartine

1 slice of your favorite bread (if gluten-free is desired, we recommend Base Culture)

Your favorite cream cheese, at room temperature (for a vegan option, we recommend Tofutti)

Lemon

Recommended Toppings

Tomato, thinly sliced

Romaine lettuce, finely shredded

Carrots, shredded

Persian cucumber, thinly sliced

Avocado, sliced

Red onion, thinly sliced

Alfalfa sprouts

Dill or chives, finely chopped

Kosher salt and freshly ground black pepper

I created this dish because it reminds me of the way I grew up eating. Shaved carrots, cucumbers, and alfalfa sprouts are all staples in the West Coast diet. I also love that you can whip up something that is a true gift to yourself, or make something for someone else that doesn't require any cooking. This is all about assembly! You can also choose your own adventure and substitute cream cheese for avocado, or take out or put in anything that speaks to you. Point is, if you were ever curious what California tasted like in the 1970s, here you go.

Toast the bread. Toast the bread lightly. Let cool.

Top. Spread the cream cheese on the toast. Layer on the toppings. We recommend this order for minimum slippage and maximum crunch: tomato, lettuce, carrots, cucumbers, avocado, red onion, and alfalfa sprouts. Squeeze on a little lemon juice, top with herbs, and season with salt and pepper.

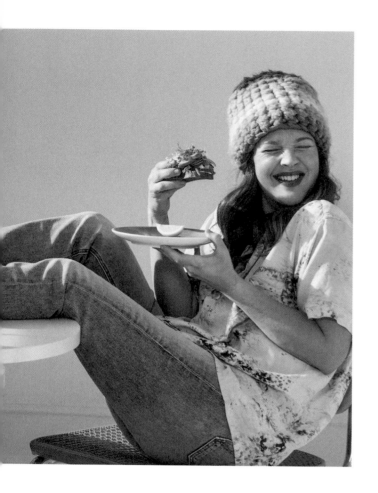
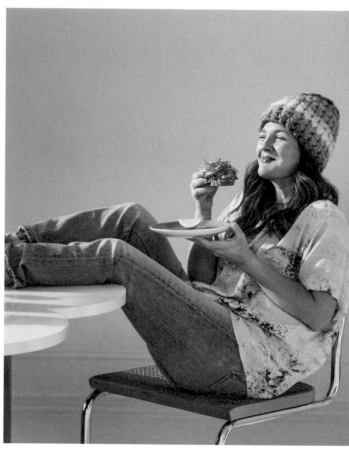

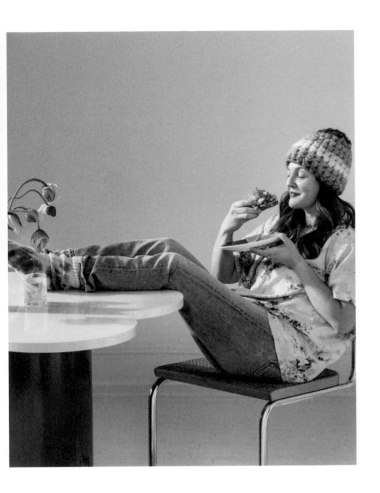

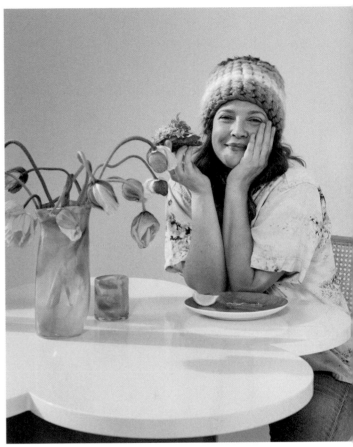

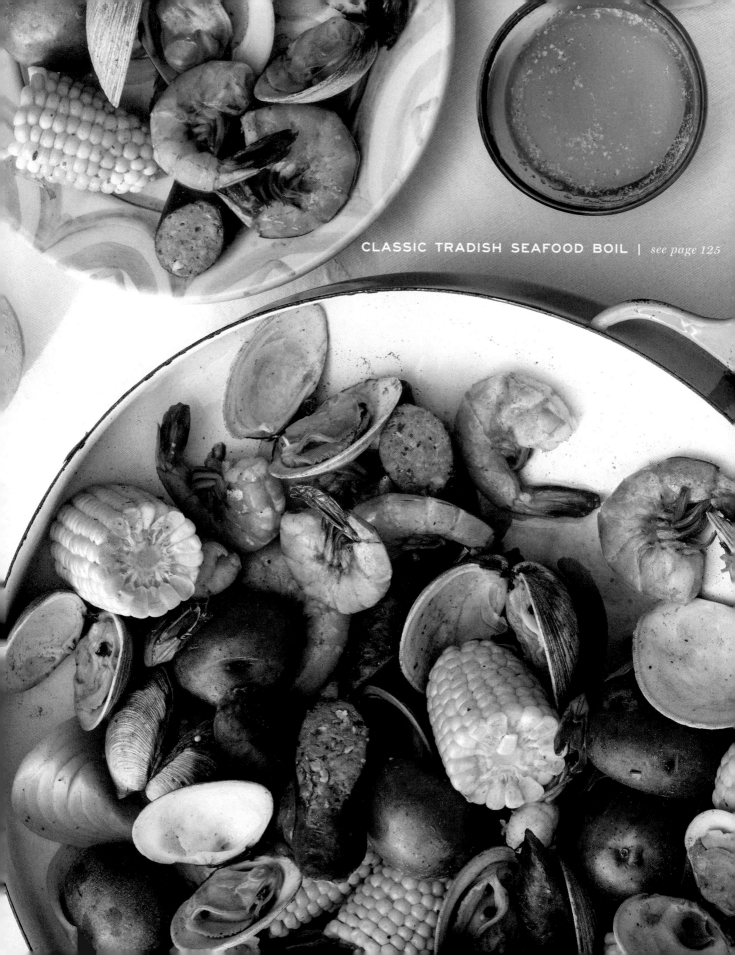

CLASSIC TRADISH SEAFOOD BOIL | *see page 125*

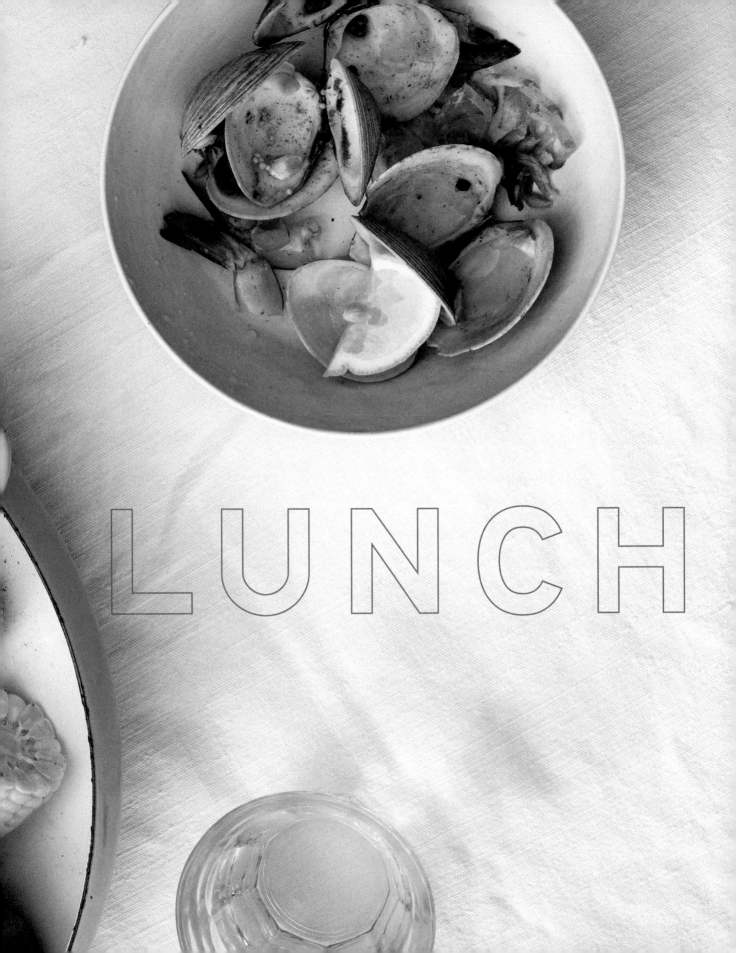

LUNCH

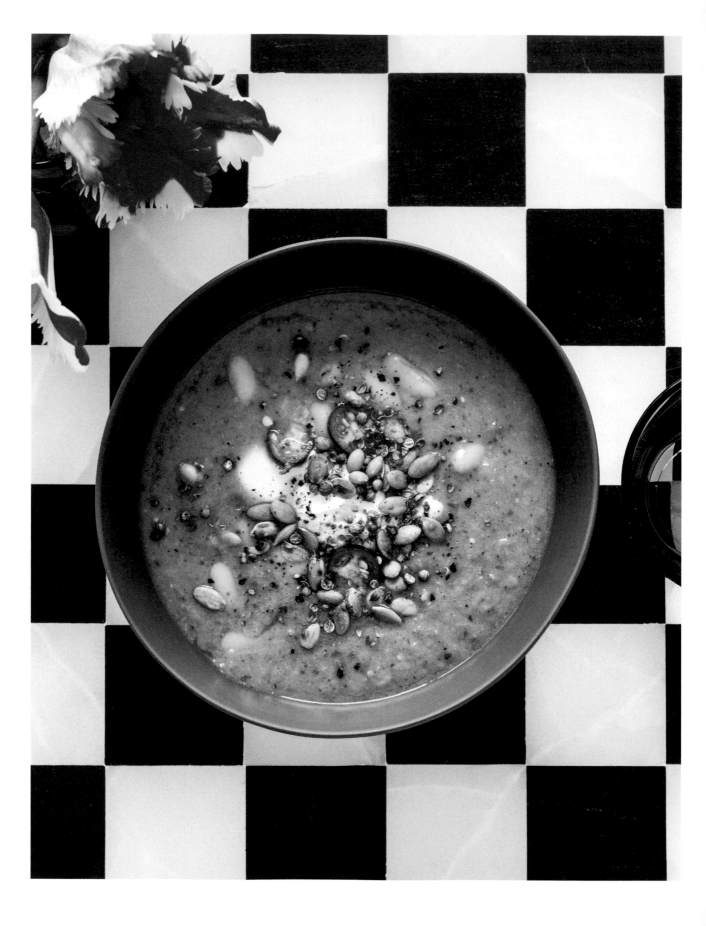

Roasted Poblano-Tomatillo Soup

MAKES 6 CUPS
SERVES 4 TO 6

4 poblano chilies

2 large or 4 small tomatillos, husks removed

4 medium shallots, unpeeled

6 large cloves garlic, unpeeled

1 jalapeño, halved lengthwise

3 tablespoons avocado oil, divided

Kosher salt and freshly ground black pepper

2 medium leeks, thinly sliced, about 2½ cups (white and light green parts only)

2 (15.5-ounce) cans cannellini beans, beans drained (and unrinsed), divided; aquafaba (bean-soaking liquid) from both cans reserved

2½ cups plus 2 tablespoons water, divided

½ cup (lightly packed) chopped cilantro (leaves and stems)

1 tablespoon freshly squeezed lime juice, plus additional lime wedges for serving

To Garnish (Optional)

Coconut yogurt

Coriander seeds, toasted and lightly crushed

Toasted pepitas

This is one of my favorite soups, and we make it often at the house. It's really a love letter to some of my favorite Mexican ingredients—poblanos, tomatillos, jalapeños, and cilantro—blended up into a wonderfully satisfying soup. There's just the right amount of heat, lovely pops of brightness from both the tomatillos and the fresh cilantro, and you can feel free to adjust the spice level by adding more (or less) jalapeño according to your preference.

Since the soup is vegan, we give it more body and a rounder mouthfeel with the use of aquafaba, the liquid from cooking the beans. So when draining the beans, don't forget to reserve the liquid from the can. (This amazing ingredient can be used as an egg or egg white substitute in many vegan recipes, too—but that's for another recipe.) You can definitely cook dry beans from scratch, but we've found that canned beans work great. The peppers and aromatics can be roasted up to 3 days in advance, and the cooked soup freezes and reheats like a dream.

Roast peppers and aromatics. Preheat the oven to 425 degrees. Place the poblanos, tomatillos, shallots, garlic, and jalapeño on a rimmed baking sheet. Drizzle with 1½ tablespoons oil. Toss to coat thoroughly and season with ½ teaspoon salt and a few grinds of black pepper. Transfer to the oven and roast until browned and caramelized, about 30 minutes, shaking the pan halfway through. Remove from the oven, being careful not to spill any of the juices released. When cool enough to handle, remove and discard the peels from the shallots and garlic as well as the stems and seeds from the poblanos and jalapeño. Set aside.

Make the base. Heat a large pot over medium-high heat. Add the remaining 1½ tablespoons oil, swirl to coat, and add the leeks. Season with salt and pepper and sauté, stirring occasionally, until softened and translucent, 4 to 5 minutes. Add 1 can of cannellini beans and the roasted peppers and aromatics, including all accumulated juices from the baking sheet, and stir.

Add 2½ cups water and all the aquafaba. Bring to a boil and then reduce heat to maintain a brisk simmer. Cook, partially covered, 10 minutes, stirring occasionally, to allow flavors to marry.

Blend the soup. Transfer the mixture to a blender and add the cilantro and lime juice. Blend until the soup is very smooth. Transfer back to the pot and add the remaining 1 can of cannellini beans. Return the heat to low to heat through. Season to taste with salt and pepper.

Serve. Transfer the hot soup to individual bowls and top with coconut yogurt and garnish with coriander seeds, toasted pepitas (if using), and a lime wedge on the side.

Coconut Fish Kilawin

For Coconut Topping

3 tablespoons unsweetened coconut chips

For the Fish

1 boneless, skinless fillet blackfish or snapper (about 8 ounces)

3 tablespoons freshly squeezed lime juice, divided, plus the zest of ½ lime

1 tablespoon plus 1 teaspoon coconut vinegar, divided

⅓ cup high-quality unsweetened coconut milk, from a well-shaken can

2 tablespoons fish sauce, plus additional for seasoning

¼ teaspoon yuzu juice (can be substituted with orange juice or additional lime juice)

½ (14-ounce) can hearts of palm, cut into ¼-inch slices (about 1 heaping cup), plus 1 teaspoon brine from can

2 teaspoons finely grated ginger

½ teaspoon minced habanero, or more to taste

½ teaspoon granulated sugar

1 small shallot, thinly sliced, rings separated

Kosher salt

I love that recipes can be so transportive, a way to learn something new about a different culture. This recipe is from the Philippines, where Pilar is from, and is near and dear to her heart.

Kilawin is basically a chilled seafood dish that is lightly "cooked" with vinegar and citrus juices—in this case lime and coconut vinegar. You can think of it like a Filipino ceviche. (Because the fish is not fully cooked, you want to take extra care and buy the freshest fish you can get your hands on.) The raw fish pieces are "kissed" by the vinegar, just marinated quickly, before being mixed with the rest of the sauce. We use coconut vinegar for this, which is mild and has a natural sweetness to it, but you can substitute it with apple cider vinegar as well.

The whole dish is rounded out by a flavorful coconut sauce—addictive and delicious!

Make the topping. In a small skillet over medium-high heat, toast the coconut chips, stirring constantly, until fragrant and lightly golden. Set aside.

Marinate the fish. Cut the fish into ¾-inch cubes. Top with 1 tablespoon lime juice and 1 teaspoon coconut vinegar. Toss gently to coat. Transfer to the refrigerator and let chill for 5 to 10 minutes.

Meanwhile, in a medium bowl whisk together the coconut milk, fish sauce, yuzu juice (or orange or lime juice if using as a substitute), hearts of palm brine, ginger, habanero, sugar, lime zest, ¼ teaspoon salt, remaining 2 tablespoons lime juice, and remaining 1 tablespoon coconut vinegar. Check for seasoning. This sauce should be a little puckery, salty and sweet, with a touch of roundness from the coconut milk. Add the marinated fish to the bowl, along with the hearts of palm and sliced shallots. Toss to coat and transfer to the refrigerator, no more than 1 hour before serving.

To serve. Taste the kilawin and season with additional fish sauce or salt, if desired. Place in a serving bowl, top with toasted coconut, and serve immediately.

Blackened Tuna with Cherry Tomato and Jicama Salsa

SERVES 2

For the Salsa

2 tablespoons freshly squeezed lime juice, from 1 to 2 limes

1 teaspoon honey

1 tablespoon cilantro stems, leaves reserved for serving

Kosher salt and freshly ground black pepper

¼ small jicama (about 3 ounces), peeled and diced into ½-inch cubes

½ cup cherry tomatoes, quartered

1 tablespoon finely chopped pickled jalapeños

For the Tuna

1 teaspoon mild chili powder

¾ teaspoon ground coriander

¾ teaspoon ground cumin

¾ teaspoon Mexican oregano

¾ teaspoon onion powder

½ teaspoon garlic powder

⅛ teaspoon ground cayenne

Kosher salt and freshly ground black pepper

1 (1½-inch-thick) ahi or yellowfin tuna steak, about 1 pound

2 teaspoons avocado oil

6 leaves butter lettuce, for serving

Fish in a lettuce cup! This dish is in heavy rotation during the summer months. Easy and delicious, I love being able to pick the whole thing up and eat it with my hands.

The spice mix can be made (and stored at room temperature) for up to 1 month in advance. We always make a double batch and use it on popcorn, salmon, and even on deviled eggs!

We serve the tuna warm in this recipe, but it's also really great cooked and chilled, and will keep in the fridge for up to 2 days. I love it with a side of Cumin-Scented Slaw (page 206).

Make the salsa. In a small bowl, whisk to combine the lime juice, honey, and cilantro stems. Season with salt and pepper. Add the jicama, cherry tomatoes, and pickled jalapeños, toss to coat, and transfer to the refrigerator until ready to serve. Can be made up to 1 day in advance.

Make the spice mix. In a small bowl, combine the chili powder, coriander, cumin, Mexican oregano, onion powder, garlic powder, cayenne, ½ teaspoon salt, and ¼ teaspoon black pepper.

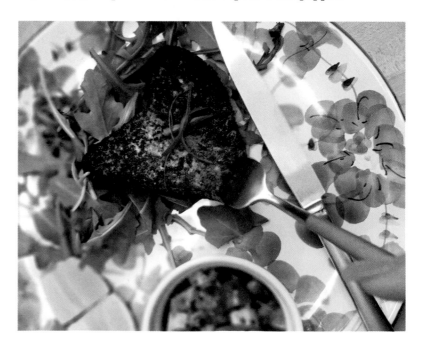

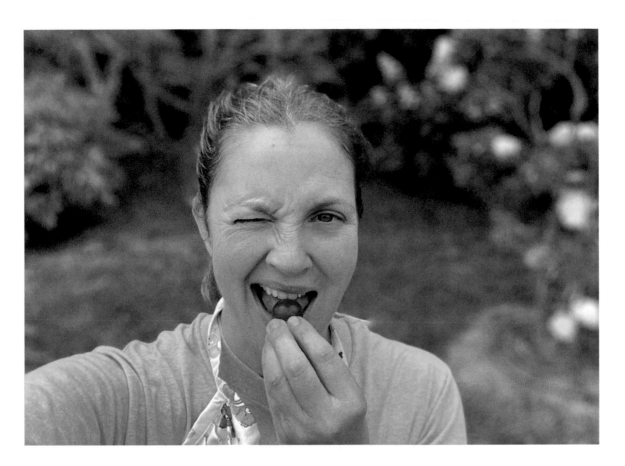

Season the tuna. Rub the tuna with the spice mix and let sit for 10 minutes at room temperature or up to 8 hours in advance, covered, in the refrigerator. (If seasoning in advance in the refrigerator, allow the tuna to sit at room temperature for 10 minutes before cooking.)

Cook. Heat a heavy-bottomed pan (such as cast-iron) over high heat. Drizzle 1 teaspoon of avocado oil on each side of the tuna. Carefully place the tuna steak on the hot pan and cook undisturbed, flipping once, halfway through cooking. For a rare steak, we recommend 3 minutes total cooking time (internal temperature of 115–120 degrees); for medium-rare, 5 minutes total cooking time (120–130 degrees); and for medium, 6 to 6½ minutes total cooking time (130–140 degrees). Remove the tuna from the pan and let rest on a cutting board for 5 minutes before slicing.

Serve. Cut the tuna against the grain into ½-inch slices. Serve in lettuce cups topped with the reserved cilantro leaves and the tomato and jicama salsa.

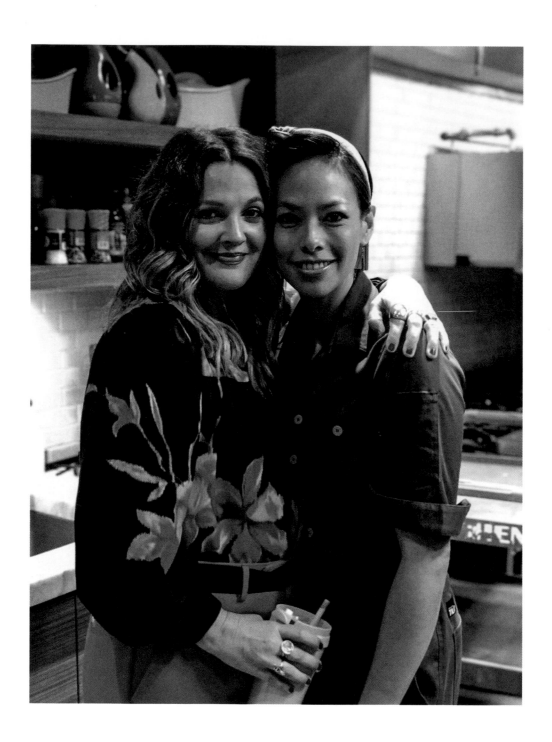

Learning to Cook with Pilar

One thing about living around the world, and really not living so much in a structured permanent home until my midtwenties, is that for years, I really wasn't good in the kitchen. I was like a takeout queen—by the way, I still love a night of takeout and a food competition show on the television. Color me happy; that is my paradise! To-go boxes and my remote control—yes, please!

When I met my cooking partner, Pilar, we bonded over Campbell's Cream of Mushroom Soup. Pilar grew up in the Philippines, and when she was sick, her mom would buy her that particular can of soup as a special treat to make her feel better. So she has very fond feelings and associations, as you can imagine! And for me, when I lived in California in the '70s, my mom used to make her famous tuna noodle casserole with Campbell's Cream of Mushroom Soup, and that flavor is synonymous with the very first dish I fell in love with. To this day, I occasionally beg my mom to make it for me—that and boxed Kraft Macaroni & Cheese, which is still my favorite food to this day.

I've been a cookbook collector ever since I was pregnant with my first daughter.

Pilar and I originally met while I was living in a New York City rental, newly divorced and pretty much flipping out and trying to just keep my head above water and survive. Pilar was a safe harbor in a storm. I was very uncomfortable in my new life. I missed California, and I was residing in a home I couldn't decorate because it wasn't really mine. I was trying to make peace with the east–west transition, not to mention the divorce or trying to get my daughter into kindergarten. I was bringing my daughters to preschool every day, raising them, and trying to stop making movies because I didn't like the hours anymore. Honestly, I just didn't really know where my life was going.

One of the things I did have was a bunch of cookbooks, which I had shipped from California to New York. I have since started a cookbook club! Okay, at that point I didn't even have a real kitchen and I couldn't cook the food, but the books were so important to me. I've been a cookbook collector ever since I was pregnant with my first daughter. The first cookbook I bought was a Williams-Sonoma one with 365 recipes for soup. Then I started buying more, and I would collect more as I traveled around the world.

Now I probably have several hundred cookbooks! And as I became more established in New York, I started to use them. Over the next two years, I spent hours in the kitchen with Pilar, cooking everything, talking about food, ingredients, interesting food seasoning combinations we both love, and flavors and details from different elements of food all over the world. When Pilar and I cook together, we like to keep it interesting and inspired. We couldn't see a vegetable or fruit without

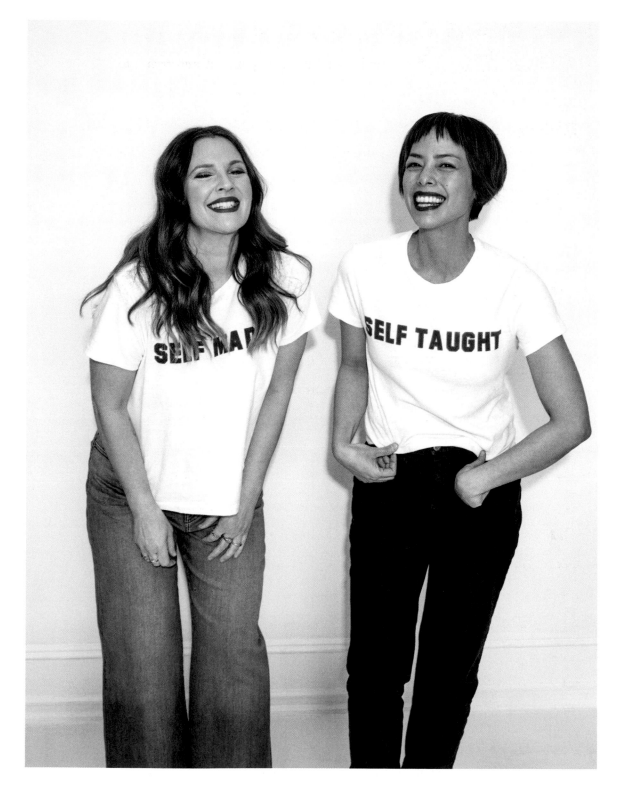

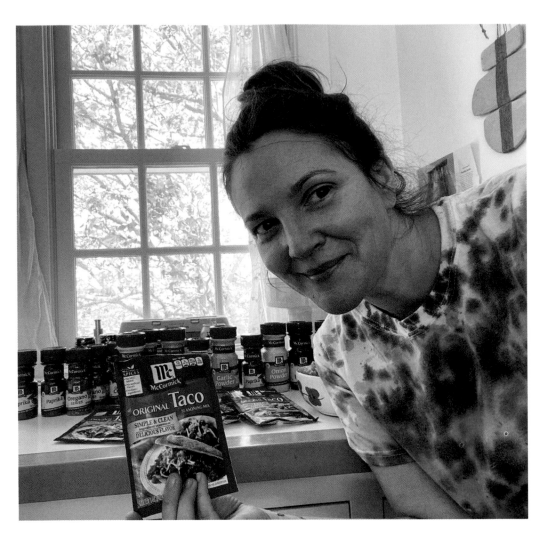

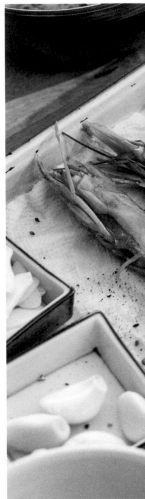

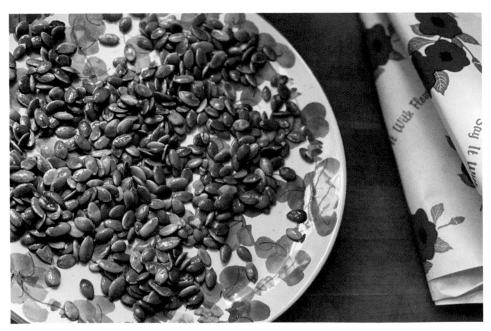

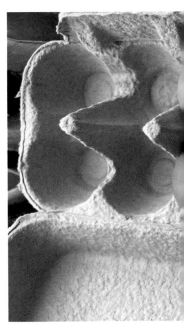

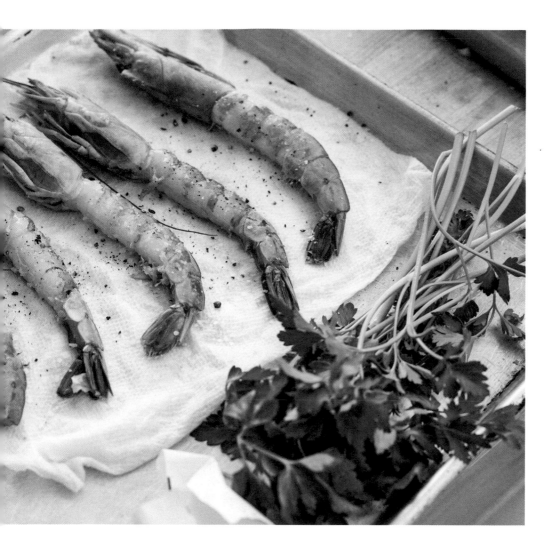

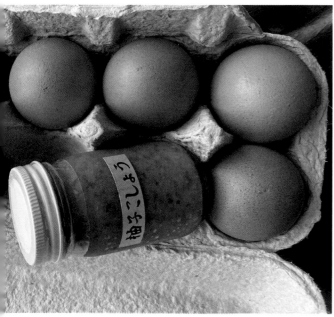

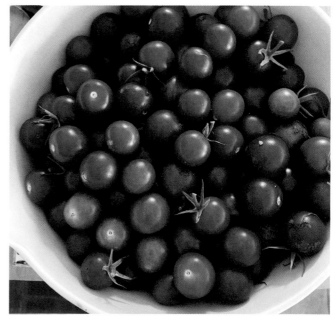

saying, "What about this flavor with that? What if you layered this blood orange with this toasted pepita? What could give food a lot of texture without a ton of carbohydrates?" I didn't want to rely on white flour for everything. Flour happens to be my favorite ingredient on the planet, and all my favorite foods are cheesy carby foods, but that's more in my comfort zone.

What I wanted was to eat food from a different locale or geographical destination every single day. And I really did want to make that happen! I think of food all the time, from the moment I wake up to the moment I sleep. If I had written this book a few years ago, I would've talked about how much I loved dinner parties and how much I thought that food was the glue that brings us all together and creates the memories. But it's funny—in the past two years, there have not been dinner parties. That is definitely a goal I have: to get back to traveling and to get back to dinner parties, lunches, anything!

But I love cooking, and I love doing it with Pilar, because we really think and feel our way through each dish, figuring out how we can make it unique, paring it down, editing it, not overcomplicating the recipes but making them feel complex and layered but still doable. And fun!

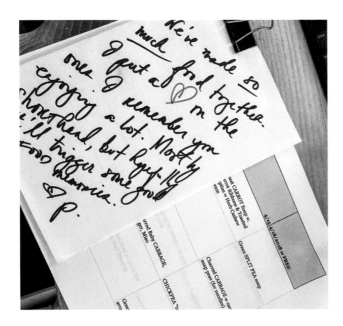

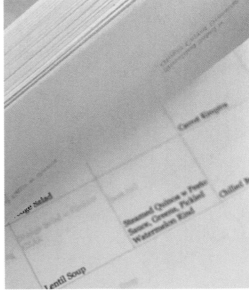

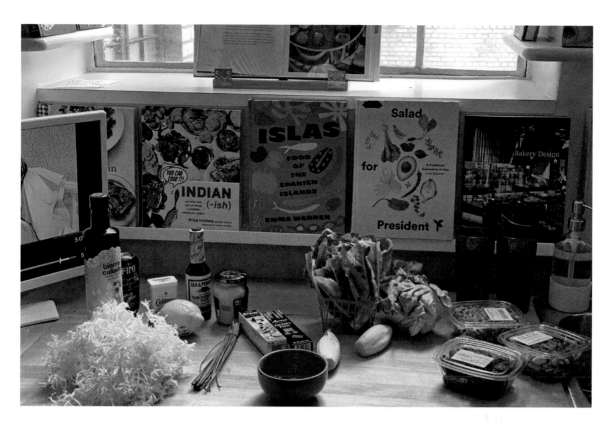

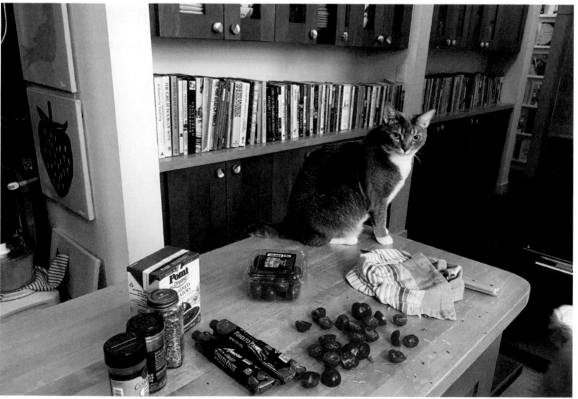

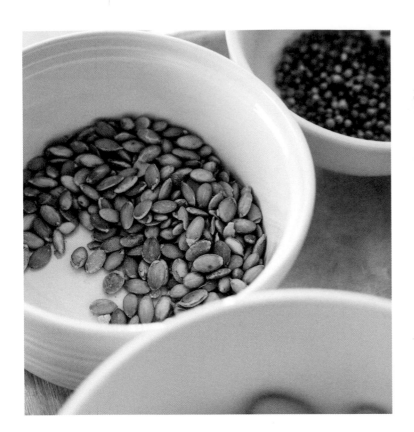

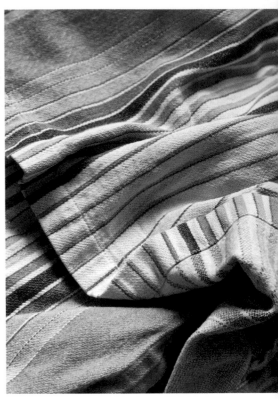

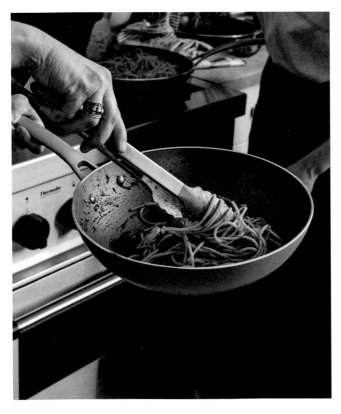

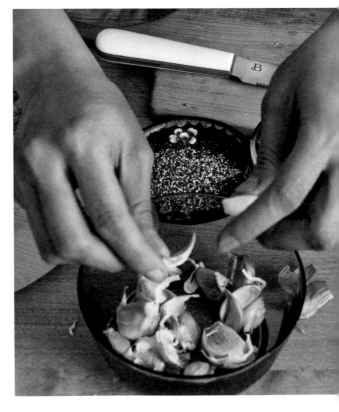

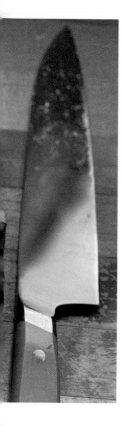

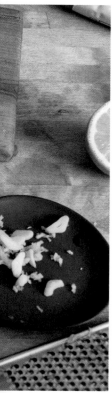

Blackened Tuna Steaks
¿ Grilled 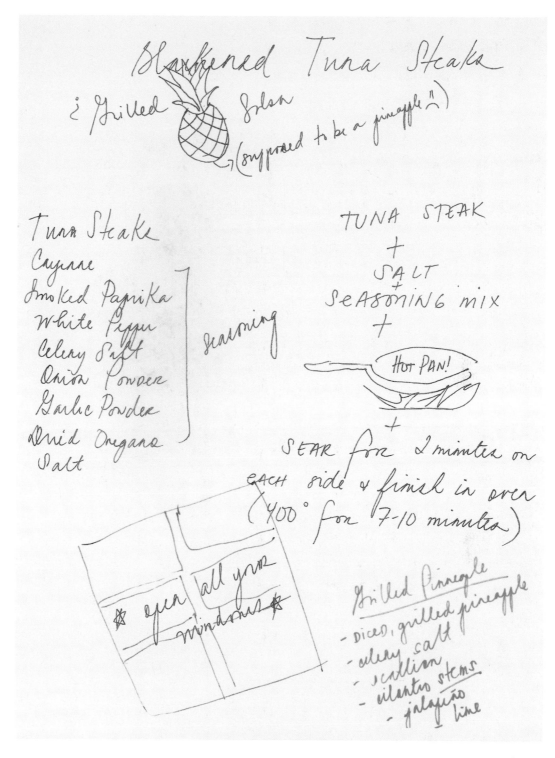 Salsa
(supposed to be a pineapple¨)

Tuna Steaks
Cayenne
Smoked Paprika   ⎤
White Pepper |
Celery Salt | seasoning
Onion Powder |
Garlic Powder |
Dried Oregano   ⎦
Salt

TUNA STEAK
+
SALT
+
SEASONING MIX
+

Hot PAN!

+
SEAR for 2 minutes on
each side & finish in oven
(400° for 7-10 minutes)

* open all your windows *

Grilled Pineapple
- diced, grilled pineapple
- celery salt
- scallion
- cilantro stems
- jalapeño   lime

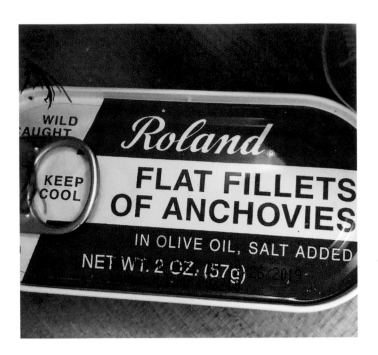

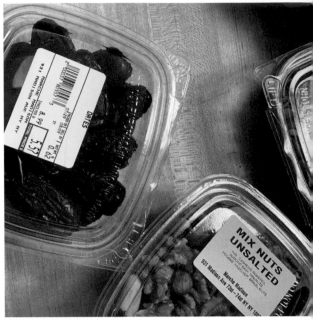

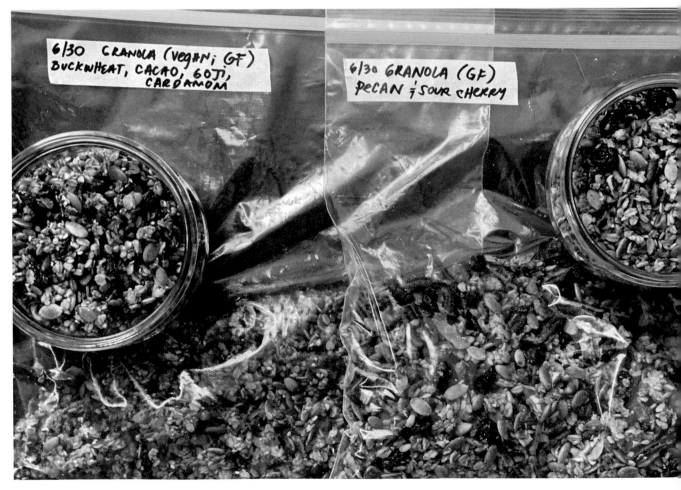

6/30 GRANOLA (VEGAN) (GF)
BUCKWHEAT, CACAO, GOJI,
CARDAMOM

6/30 GRANOLA (GF)
PECAN & SOUR CHERRY

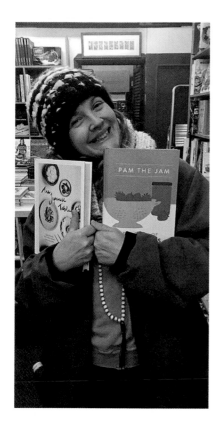

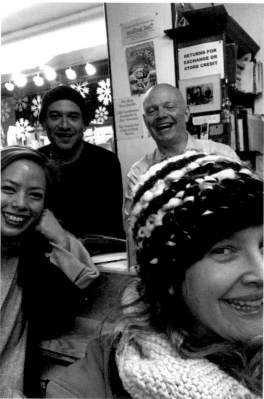

When I think about it, I've learned more from authentic street food than I have from fancy restaurants. Which reinforces my feeling about wanting to come to this book with a real approach and knowledge and passion, but also jumble it all up with Pilar's incredible self-taught skills. That's another thing I love about Pilar—she's self-taught, just like me. Sometimes I rebel when people have an overly professional outlook; sometimes they can be a little full of boundaries and rules and guidelines. Pilar and I aren't like that! We like to play, we like to paint, we like to let loose and express ourselves. I am self-made—I literally have been self-generating my entire life—if I waited for a job, it wouldn't come. And Pilar has empowered me to feel like I can make delicious things in the kitchen, and I'm so grateful and excited to now share that feeling with everyone.

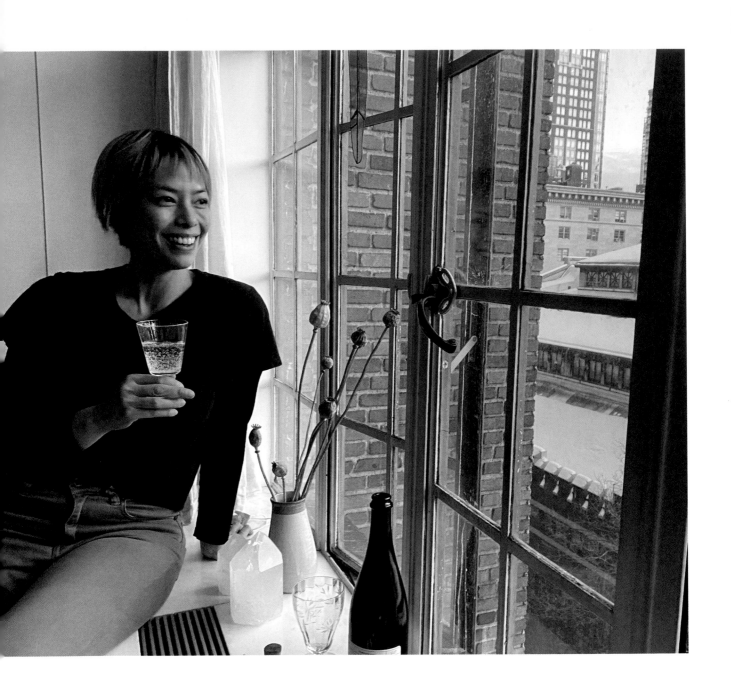

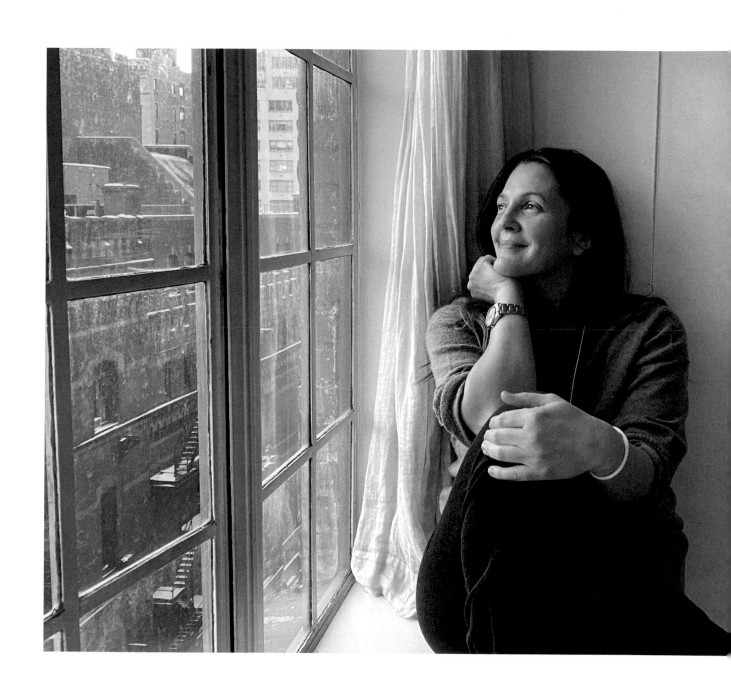

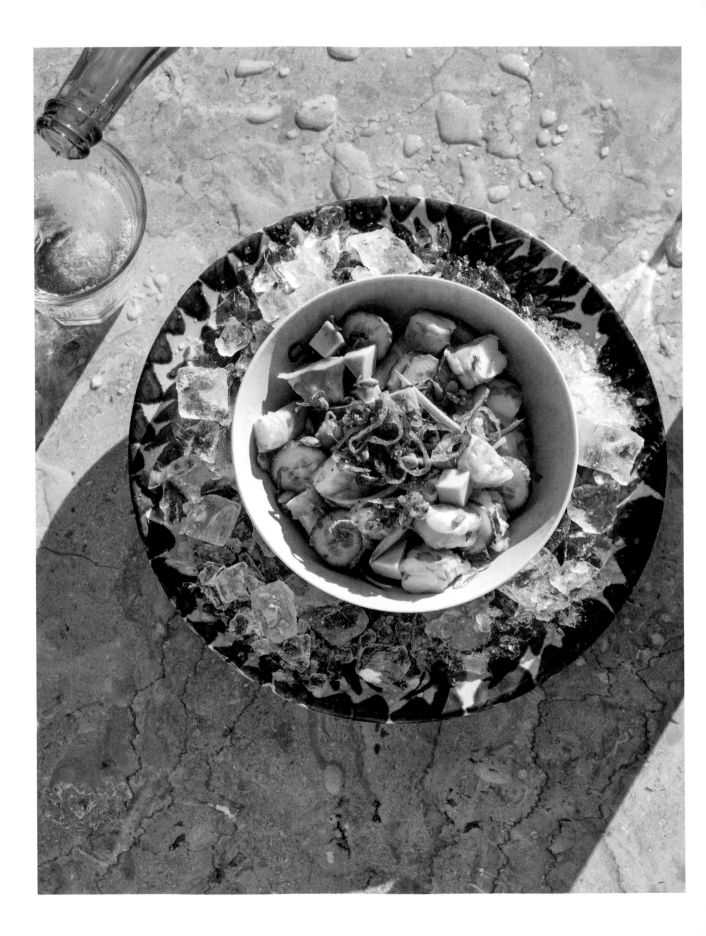

Shrimp Ceviche with Lime, Red Onion, and Cilantro

1 medium red onion

1 pound (21/25) shell-on shrimp, backs split and inner tract removed

5 cloves garlic, unpeeled and smashed

½ bunch cilantro, tied into a bundle with kitchen string, plus ¼ cup finely chopped cilantro stems, divided

1 bay leaf

Kosher salt

2 teaspoons black peppercorns

¼ cup freshly squeezed lime juice from about 2 limes, plus additional lime wedges for serving

1 teaspoon fish sauce

1 Persian cucumber, thinly sliced into half moons

1 Roma tomato, seeded and diced

1 serrano or habanero pepper, seeded and chopped (optional)

1 avocado, peeled, pitted, and cut into ½-inch cubes

(ingredients continue)

Talk about recipes being transportive! This recipe makes us think of being in the sun (by a pool! at a beach!) with a bag of chips, toes in the water.

We absolutely love this recipe, which has great contrast in texture and in flavor—the sweet pops of plump shrimp, the creaminess of the avocado, the crunch from the cucumber—just a whole lot of yum.

Poaching the shrimp starting with cold water is a great little tip; this ensures a gentler cook that won't overcook or toughen up your shrimp.

We actually love the idea of serving this dish side by side with the Coconut Fish Kilawin (page 77) for a little ceviche party.

Poach the shrimp. Prepare an ice bath and set aside. Slice the red onion into 6 wedges lengthwise. Set aside 1 wedge for later. In a medium pot, combine the shrimp, 5 onion wedges, garlic, cilantro bundle, and bay leaf. Cover with cold water, just to the top of the shrimp. Add 1 tablespoon of salt and black peppercorns and place over medium-low heat. Heat until the liquid is just about to simmer, 13 to 15 minutes.

Check for doneness. Remove one shrimp and check for doneness: it should be completely opaque, center to edge, and with a bit of bounce. If not fully cooked, return the shrimp to the hot liquid and check every 30 seconds, until cooked through. Using a slotted spoon, transfer all the shrimp to the prepared ice bath. Set aside the poaching liquid for the dressing.

Let the shrimp chill for 1 minute in the ice bath, and then immediately drain to ensure as much flavor as possible is retained, and that the shrimp do not get waterlogged. Peel the shrimp and slice in ¾-inch pieces.

Dress the shrimp. Measure 3 tablespoons poaching liquid and add to a small bowl. Add the lime juice, fish sauce, and cilantro stems. Add the shrimp, toss to coat, and season to taste with salt or fish sauce. Transfer the bowl to the refrigerator to chill thoroughly, at least 30 minutes and up to 6 hours in advance.

For Pepita Crunch (Optional)

2 tablespoons avocado oil

2 medium shallots, peeled and thinly sliced crosswise (1 heaping cup)

¼ cup raw pepitas

Flaky sea salt (we love Maldon)

Finely grated zest of 1 lime

Finely slice the remaining red onion wedge lengthwise and place the slices in a small bowl filled with ice water.

Make the pepita crunch (optional). Heat a medium skillet over medium heat and add the avocado oil. When oil is shimmering, add the shallots. Fry, stirring continuously, until golden and nearly crisp, 9 to 10 minutes. Add pepitas and continue to cook, stirring, until the seeds are toasted and shallots are deeply caramelized and crispy throughout, about 2 minutes more. Remove to a paper towel–lined plate and season with flaky sea salt and lime zest. Let cool thoroughly and transfer to a cutting board. Coarsely chop.

Serve. Just before serving, drain the iced red onion slices. Add to the shrimp mixture, along with the cucumber, tomato, chilies (if using), and avocado. Fold to combine and divide among serving bowls, topped with Pepita Crunch and additional lime wedges on the side.

Japchae (Sweet Potato Noodles with Sesame, Spinach, and Carrots)

MAKES 6 CUPS
SERVES 4

8 ounces sweet potato glass noodles

3 tablespoons sesame oil, divided, plus additional for serving

1 tablespoon agave syrup

5 tablespoons tamari (or soy sauce if not keeping gluten-free)

¼ cup plus 1 tablespoon rice wine vinegar

½ cup water

3 tablespoons toasted sesame seeds, plus additional for serving

2 scallions, thinly sliced, white and green parts separated

1 large yellow onion, thinly sliced

2 ounces bean sprouts, rinsed

Kosher salt

5 ounces shredded carrots

2 tablespoons mirin, divided

1 medium bunch flat-leaf spinach, rinsed, roughly chopped

2 large eggs

Freshly ground black pepper

I love love love all noodles, in every single shape and size—and Korean dangmyeon, or sweet potato glass noodles, are no exception. If you've never had them before, imagine a fat glass noodle, a little thicker and longer than a strand of spaghetti, that is slippery and chewy when cooked. Part of the fun when cooking these is that you have to take a pair of scissors to them, after they're boiled, to cut them into more manageable lengths. If not, you'll be forever like Lady and the Tramp (with no kiss). Sweet potato noodles can be found in most East Asian grocery stores or ordered online.

Japchae is a Korean stir-fried noodle dish that's loaded with tons of vegetables, sesame, and scallions (just a few of my favorite things).

A little salty, a little sweet, this dish is great for a gathering, as it's a definite crowd-pleaser. It's just as tasty hot as it is at room temperature, but it also keeps really well in the fridge for up to three days.

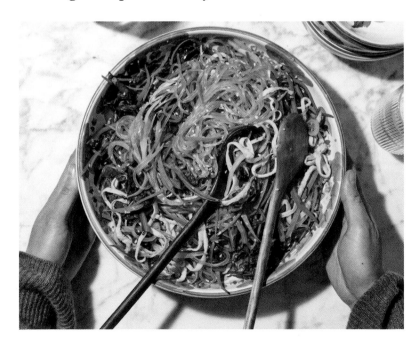

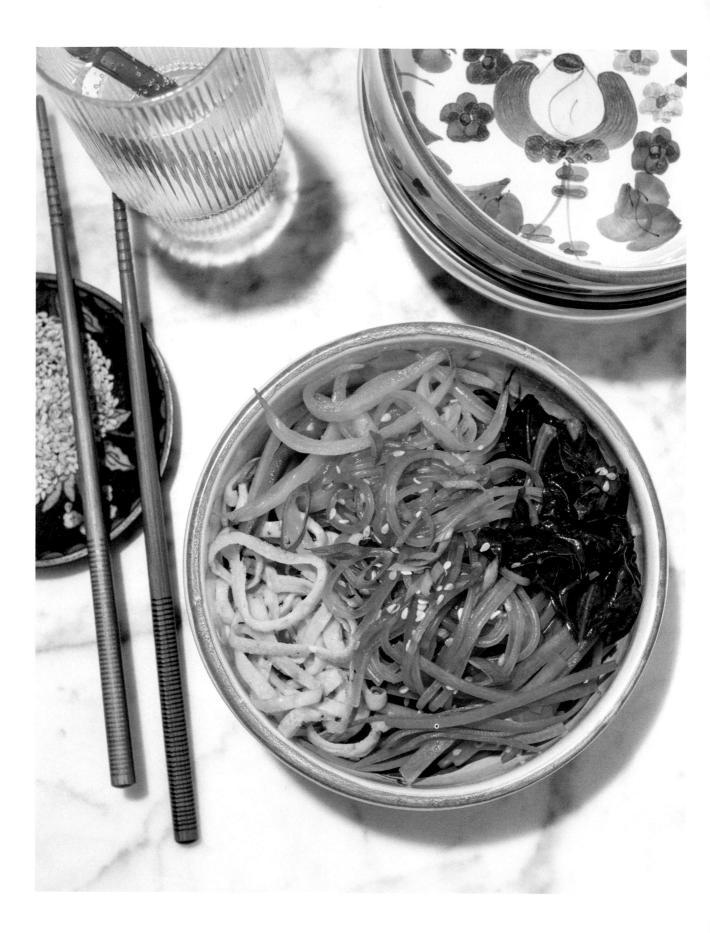

Cook the noodles. Place a large pot of water over high heat and bring to a boil. Add the sweet potato glass noodles and return to a boil. Cook until the noodles are tender and springy, about 6 minutes. Drain and rinse in cold water to stop the cooking. Transfer to a large bowl and, using kitchen shears, make 5 or 6 snips into the pile of noodles to shorten them into 6- or 7-inch pieces.

In a large nonstick skillet, combine 1½ tablespoons of the sesame oil with the agave syrup, tamari, vinegar, and water. Bring to a boil over medium-high heat. Add the noodles and toss until well coated. Continue to cook over medium-high heat, stirring constantly. The noodles will go from translucent to glossy and amber-hued as they begin to absorb the sauce, about 1 minute. As soon as they turn glossy, remove from the heat, transfer the noodles and the remaining sauce back to the large bowl, add the sesame seeds and scallion whites, and mix to distribute. Set aside. Wipe out the skillet.

Prepare the vegetable and egg topping. Return the skillet and set over high heat. Add 1 tablespoon sesame oil, swirl to coat, and add the onions and bean sprouts. Season with salt and sauté, stirring occasionally, until onions begin to soften, about 2 minutes. Add the carrots, cook for another 30 seconds, and add 1 tablespoon mirin, stirring the bottom of the skillet to deglaze. Remove the contents of the skillet to a bowl and add the remaining 1 tablespoon of mirin and spinach to the pan. Cook, stirring, until the spinach is barely wilted, about 30 seconds to 1 minute. Remove from the heat and transfer to the bowl with onions and carrots. Wipe out the skillet, and set over medium heat.

Whisk the eggs in a medium bowl and season with salt and pepper. Add the remaining 1½ teaspoons sesame oil to the skillet and swirl to coat. Add the eggs, tilting the skillet so that uncooked egg can fill the empty parts of the pan, as if you are making a very large, thin pancake. Continue cooking, reducing the heat if necessary to prevent browning, until the egg is nearly cooked on top, about 2 minutes. Transfer to a cutting board, roll the egg into a cigar, and slice into thin strips.

Serve. Pile the noodles into a bowl and surround with vegetables and egg strips. Top with additional sesame seeds and scallion greens, plus a drizzle of sesame oil.

Spiced Spaghetti Squash Patties

MAKES 8 (3-INCH) PATTIES
AND 1¼ CUPS RAITA

SERVES 4

For the Patties

1 small spaghetti squash,
about 2 pounds

Kosher salt and freshly
ground black pepper

2 tablespoons plus 2
teaspoons olive oil, divided

Heaping ½ cup cooked
white quinoa

⅔ cup frozen peas

3 tablespoons finely chopped
cilantro stems (leaves saved
for raita, recipe follows)

2 teaspoons tamarind paste,
or 1 tablespoon brown sugar
plus juice of ½ lime

2 tablespoons chickpea flour

1½ teaspoons curry powder

1 teaspoon garam masala

¾ teaspoon fennel seed

½ teaspoon ground turmeric

¼ teaspoon red pepper
flakes

Spaghetti squash, like cooked beans and roasted sweet potatoes, are things we love to cook ahead and have on hand to incorporate into dishes. Because spaghetti squash doesn't have a very powerful flavor, it is a great base for these South Asian–inspired spiced patties; they remind me of one of my favorite things: Indian samosas. This dish is packed with a *ton* of spices that play very well together. If you're in a bit of a rut with some of your regular spices, this is the recipe for you.

The patties cook up to a beautiful golden color, thanks to the turmeric, garam masala, and curry. A quick note: let the patties cool slightly after cooking as they will be very delicate hot out of the oven. They firm up as they cool.

The formed, raw patties can be frozen up to one month, making them an easy grab-and-cook option for a weeknight meal.

Roast spaghetti squash. Preheat the oven to 375 degrees. Line a rimmed baking sheet with parchment paper. Cut the spaghetti squash in half lengthwise. Scoop out the seeds and discard. Season the flesh side of the squash with salt and pepper and a drizzle of

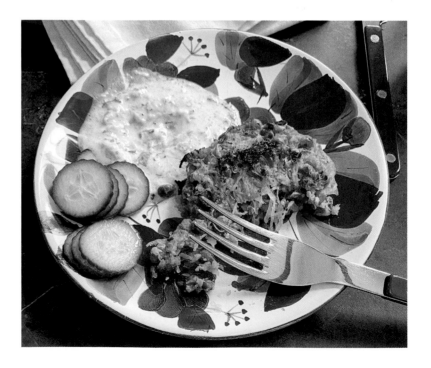

For the Raita

2 Persian cucumbers, finely grated, plus additional, sliced and salted, for serving

Kosher salt and freshly ground black pepper

1 cup plain yogurt (for a vegan option, we recommend Tofutti sour cream, thinned with 1 tablespoon water)

1 clove garlic, peeled and grated

½ teaspoon ground cumin

1 tablespoon freshly squeezed lemon juice, plus zest of 1 lemon

2 tablespoons (lightly packed) finely chopped mint

2 tablespoons (lightly packed) finely chopped cilantro leaves

½ teaspoon olive oil

Lemon wedges, for serving

olive oil, and place cut-side down on the prepared baking sheet. Transfer to the oven and roast for about 30 minutes until there is little resistance when the skin is pierced with a paring knife. Remove the squash from the oven and let cool completely.

Using a fork, scrape the squash into strands and measure about 2½ cups, lightly packed. Squeeze the spaghetti squash to expel any excess liquid and transfer to a large bowl. Reserve the remaining spaghetti squash for another use. (Cooked spaghetti squash can be made ahead and stored in an airtight container in the refrigerator for up to 5 days.)

Make the patties. Raise the oven temperature to 400 degrees.

Add the quinoa to the bowl with the spaghetti squash, along with the peas, cilantro stems, and tamarind paste. Sprinkle on the chickpea flour, curry powder, garam masala, fennel seed, turmeric, red pepper flakes, 1¼ teaspoons salt, and ¼ teaspoon pepper. Gently fold until thoroughly combined.

Using a 3-inch ring mold, or ½-cup measuring cup, form 8 patties (a scant ½ cup each) on a parchment-lined baking sheet, packing the mixture firmly before unmolding. The patties will be very tender at this point. Transfer the baking sheet to the freezer and freeze until the patties are slightly firm, about 20 minutes.

Cook the patties. Preheat a skillet over medium-high heat. Add 1 tablespoon of olive oil and swirl to coat. Add 4 patties and cook until browned and crisp in spots, flipping once, 1 to 1½ minutes per side, adjusting the heat as necessary to prevent overbrowning. Transfer the patties to the baking sheet and repeat with the remaining patties. Place the baking sheet in the oven and bake until the patties are warmed through, 10 to 12 minutes. Remove from the oven and let sit for 3 to 5 minutes, to allow the patties to firm up.

Make the raita. In a medium bowl, toss the cucumber with ½ teaspoon salt and let sit for 5 minutes. Drain as much cucumber water as possible, squeezing the grated cucumber to expel excess liquid. Add the yogurt (or vegan sour cream), garlic, ground cumin, lemon juice, lemon zest, mint, cilantro, and olive oil. Mix to combine and season to taste with salt and pepper.

Serve. Serve warm patties with a side of raita, additional salted cucumber slices, and lemon wedges.

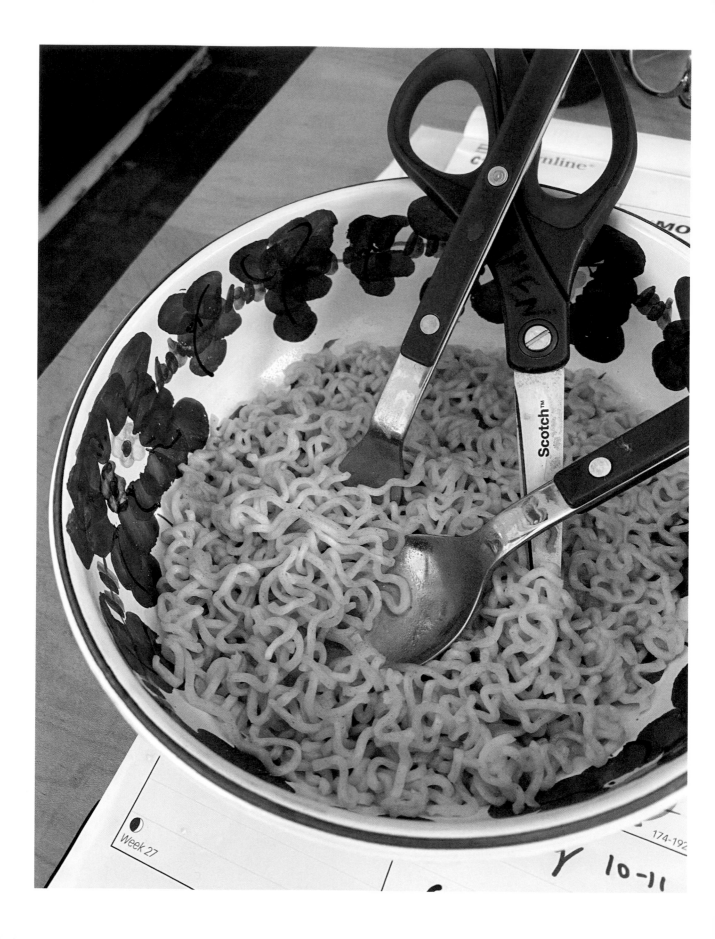

Ramen Scissors!

Pilar: One of the reasons I love Frankie and Olive's Roast Chicken (page 173) is that we try to make it once a week at the house. It's about really trying to create that ritual with your daughters. I mean, sometimes they like it; sometimes they don't!

Drew: That makes me think of a memory from during the shutdown. I bought them Top Ramen, and they had seen this thing—probably on TikTok—and asked me to give them a pair of scissors. I did and they ate their ramen with scissors, cutting the noodles out of their mouths. I felt like it became their favorite meal during the shutdown—ramen scissors night. Because they were so happy.

Pilar: And they're going to remember that! Years from now, they'll be on the floor, laughing about the ramen scissors night.

Drew: We baked so much during the shutdown. I've been giving my kids the flour and the bowl and the eggs—I've had so many disasters in the kitchen that were just the most beautiful messes I've ever seen, watching kids bake. I've since tried to get more organized about it, because it was just so much chaos.

When I was pregnant with Olive, I made the grilled cheese sandwich that's in this book, just for myself at first. I started cooking then because I thought, I'm going to have to make food for this baby at some point; I'd better start practicing. And I got that Williams-Sonoma cookbook *Soup of the Day*. I was hot as hell in one of the hottest summers in California on record, like eight months pregnant, trying to make hot soup, sweating my ass off! It did not look the way it was supposed to in my head . . .

I started with soups, with one pot. I'm not good at multitasking. I'm a focused one-dish person.

Pilar: Your kids are so, so clearly cut from your cloth in terms of their preferences. The stuff you gravitate to is so varied. Frankie has a very particular stream—she loves all the crunchy crunchies. The chickpeas, the iceberg lettuce. She loves her Cholula, just like her mom.

Drew: I love the Cholula! I won't eat without the Cholula!

Pilar: And Olive loves the bread, and the mayonnaise, and all that good stuff!

Drew: It's all white foods with Olive. It's so hard to get her out of the beige circle. Quesadillas, grilled cheese . . .

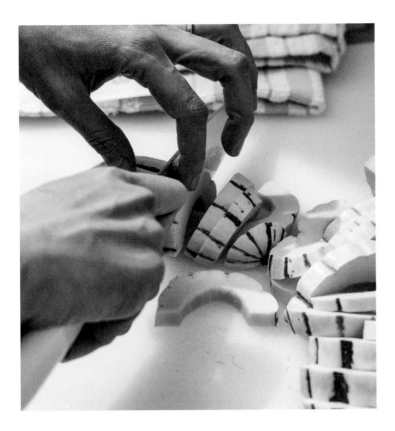

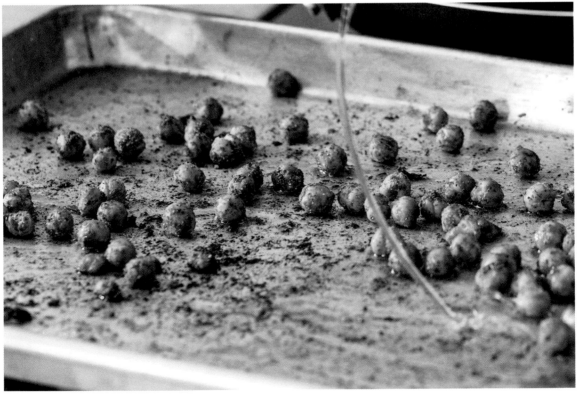

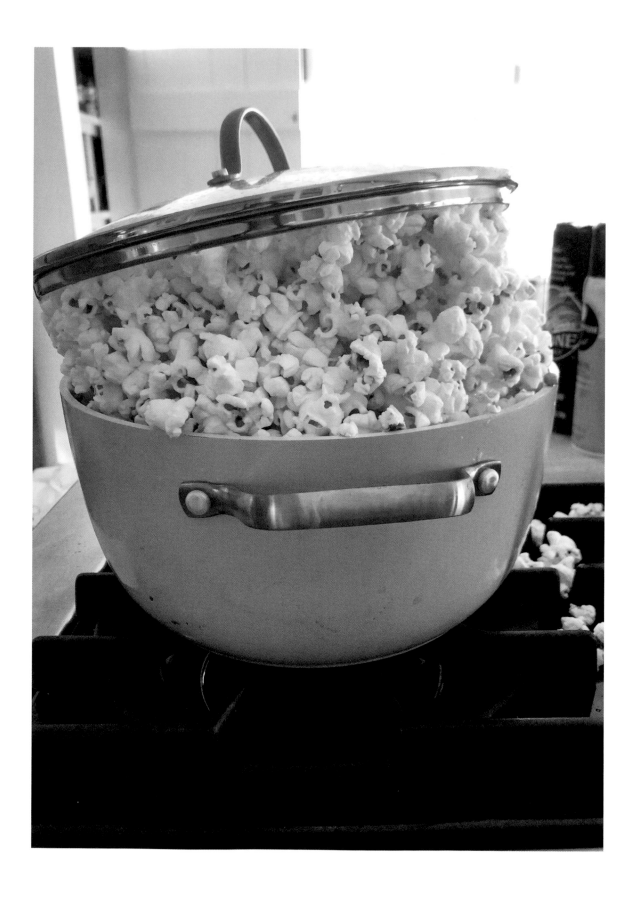

Pilar: Olive does love those broccoli bites, just like you do. That was something I had made for them, and they were nervous to try them. And then you said, "Oh, I really like these!" and now Olive eats them, too! They surprise us sometimes.

Drew: It's a miracle. I love those broccoli bites so much.

I think you become a cook when you have kids, and you try to make these elaborate meals for them, colorful and balanced . . . And then they fill their bellies with buttered pasta or popcorn. You try to get them to try new things, and then you think that one of their favorite meals was the ramen scissors night from the shutdown.

Pilar: But when they're really joyful and eating something you've made for them, it feels like the most victorious win ever.

Drew: The biggest win ever!

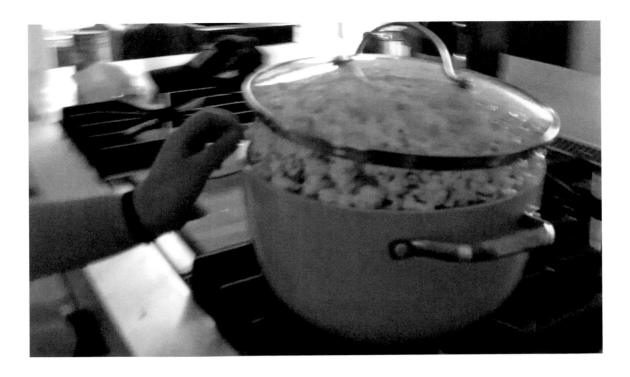

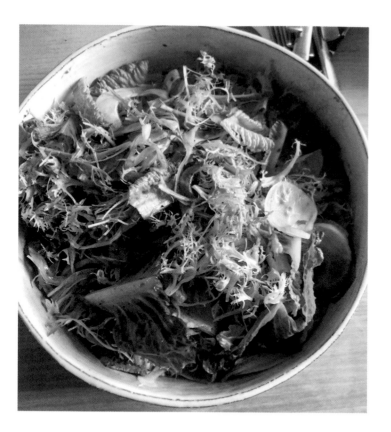

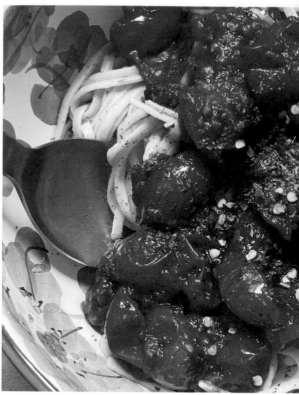

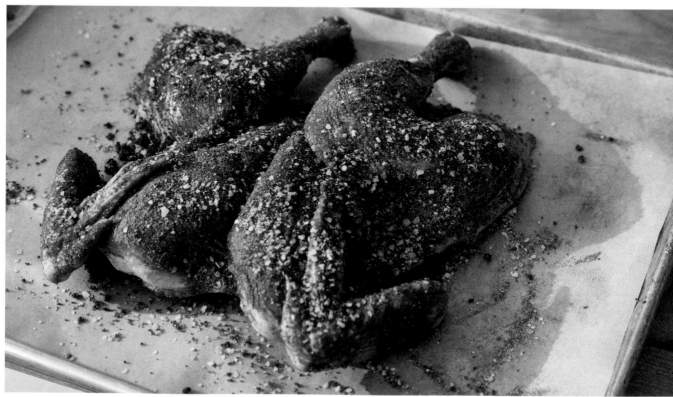

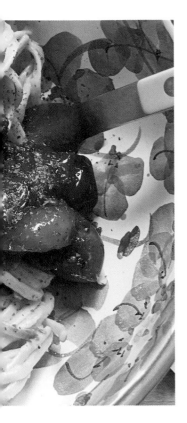

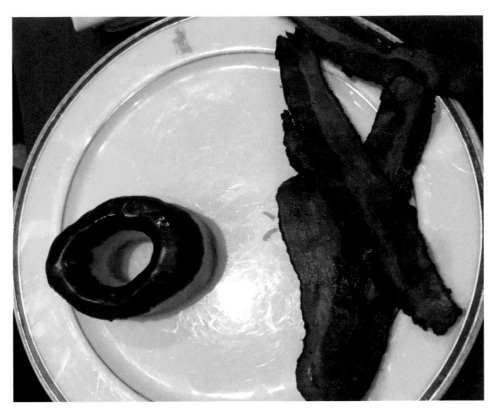

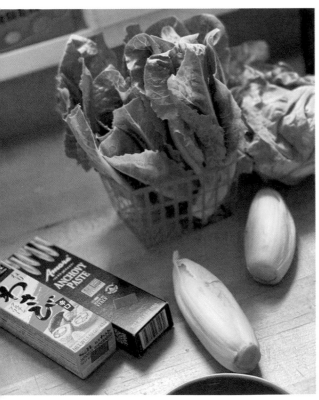

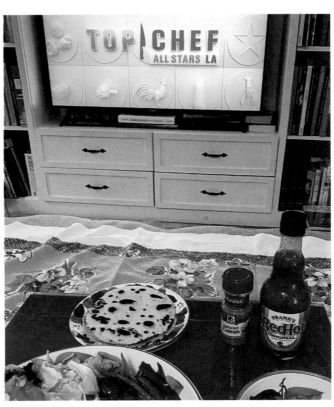

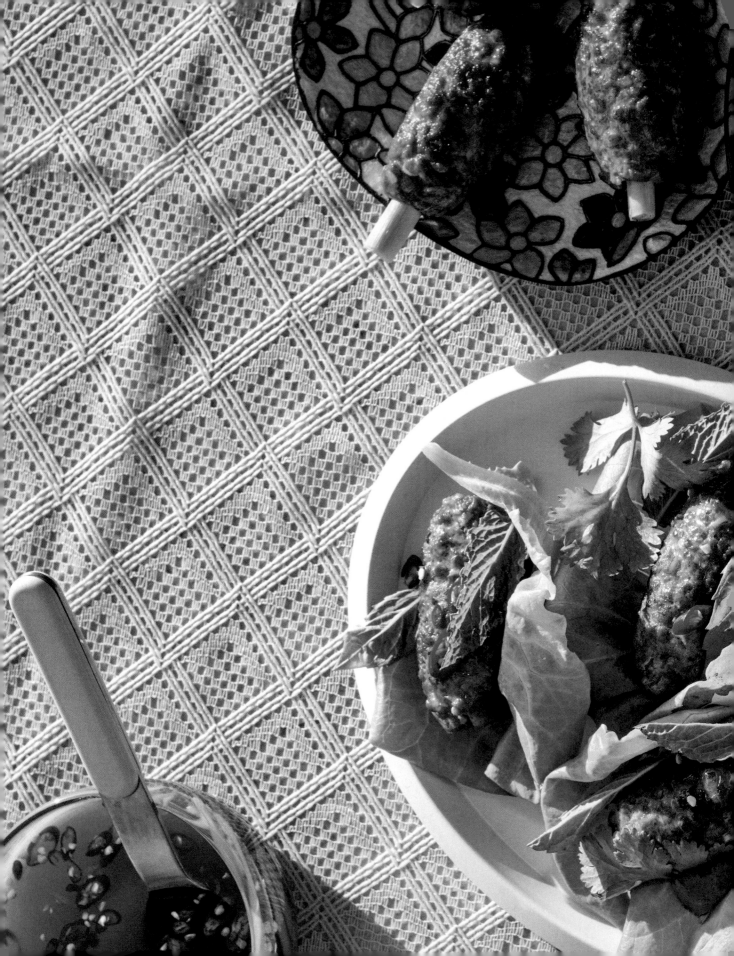

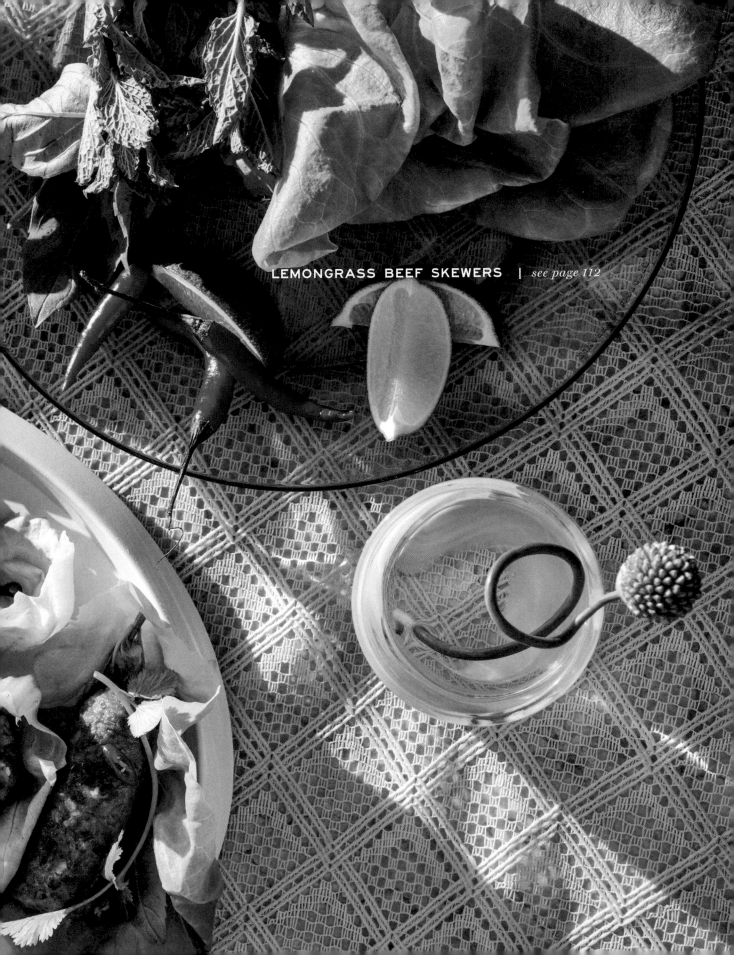

LEMONGRASS BEEF SKEWERS | *see page 112*

Lemongrass Beef Skewers

4 lemongrass stalks

1 large lime leaf, finely chopped, or zest of 2 limes

1 scallion, green and white parts, thinly sliced crosswise

2 tablespoons finely chopped cilantro stems, plus cilantro leaves reserved for serving

1 small shallot, finely chopped (1 heaping tablespoon)

1 tablespoon fish sauce

½ tablespoon curry powder

1 pound (85% lean) ground beef

1½ teaspoons coconut oil, divided, plus additional as necessary for searing

12 Thai basil or Italian basil leaves for skewers, plus additional for serving

12 butter lettuce leaves, for serving, if desired

Mint, for serving

Lime wedges, for serving

Nuoc Cham, for serving (recipe follows)

I absolutely love this recipe! These fragrant skewers are real crowd-pleasers, and I promise they're as easy to make as your favorite meatballs.

We took inspiration from Vietnamese bò lá lốt, parcels of seasoned beef wrapped in betel leaves and grilled over charcoal. Drool! Instead of betel leaves, we use basil leaves—which are much easier to source—while still tipping our hat to some of the original flavors of curry, fish sauce, and lemongrass. If you can get your hands on Thai basil and lime leaves, great, but if not, they can be easily (and deliciously) substituted with lime zest and Italian basil.

For this recipe, we are cooking on the stovetop, but I think they would be really delicious if you took them outside and cooked them on the grill.

Salty, sweet, sour, and just a little funky—a delicious party in your mouth.

These can be made ahead, and the fully assembled (raw) skewers can be frozen for up to 1 month.

Make the spiced beef mix. Finely mince 1 stalk of lemongrass, to measure 2 tablespoons. In a large bowl, combine the minced lemongrass, lime leaves (or lime zest), scallion, cilantro stems, shallots, fish sauce, and curry powder. Stir to combine. Add the ground beef, and using your hands or a wooden spoon, mix until thoroughly combined. Be careful not to overmix or the skewers will be tough. (The spiced beef mixture can be made up to 2 days ahead. Keep in an airtight container in the refrigerator until ready to use.)

Check for seasoning. We always recommend cooking off a small portion of the mixture first, to check the taste and make any last-minute flavor adjustments. It should taste well seasoned and fragrant with a variety of notes and aromas—salty, sweet, sour, and funky. Heat ½ teaspoon of coconut oil in a skillet and sear a small piece of the mixture until golden and cooked through. Taste and adjust the beef mixture with additional fish sauce or spices to suit your palate.

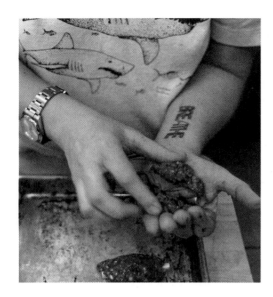

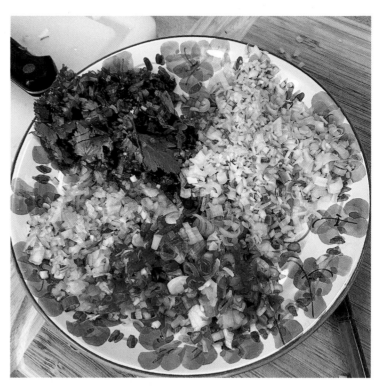

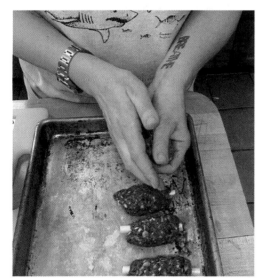

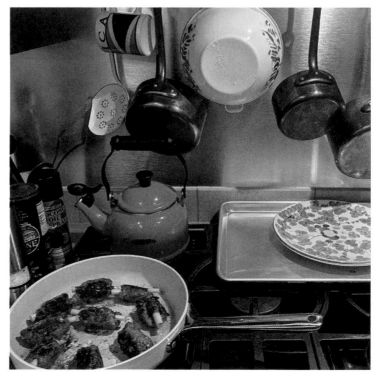

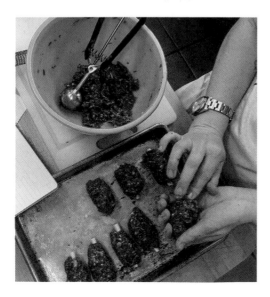

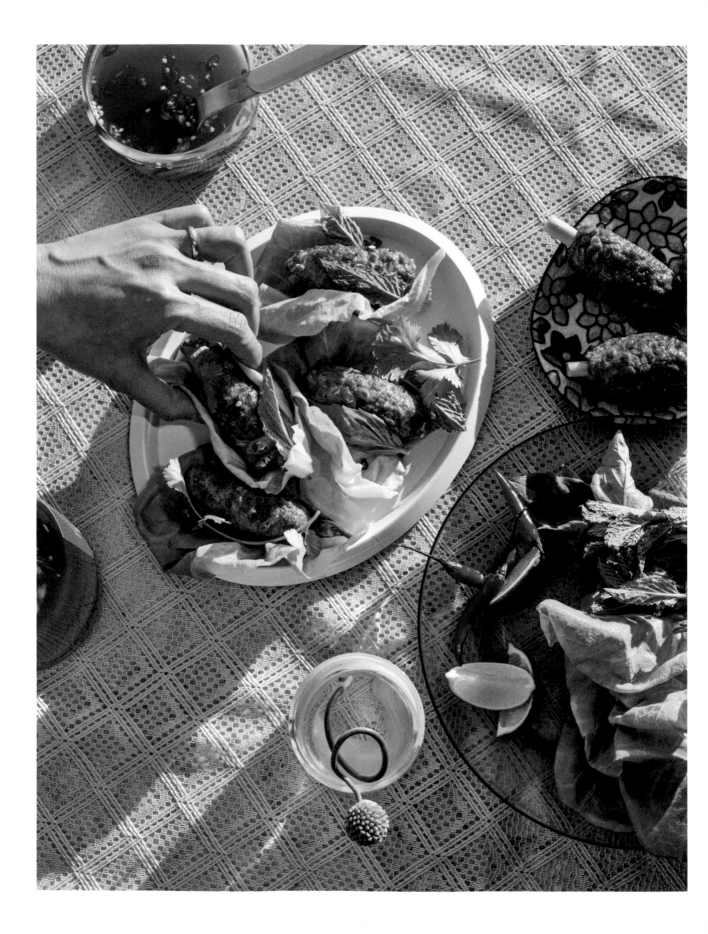

Form the skewers. Cut each of the remaining 3 lemongrass stalks into 4 skewers (12 pieces total). Divide the beef mixture into 12 equal portions, roughly 3 tablespoons each. (We use a mini ice cream scoop to help things along.) Roll each portion into a 2-inch log. Make a lengthwise indent with your index finger. Take a lemongrass skewer, wrap a piece of basil around it, and place it into the indentation. Pinch the meat to seal (rolling it between your palms also helps) so that the basil is fully enclosed, and the skewer looks something like a lollipop. Repeat with the remaining 11 portions. (Skewers can be fully assembled and frozen up to 1 month. Defrost in the refrigerator overnight before cooking.)

Cook. Heat a large, heavy-bottomed pan (like a cast-iron skillet) over medium-high heat. Add 1 teaspoon coconut oil and swirl to coat. Gently add skewers, making sure not to overcrowd the pan (you may have to work in batches). Sear each side until deeply golden and just cooked through, about 8 minutes total. (That's 4 sides at 2 minutes apiece.)

To finish. Serve skewers with a side of lettuce, basil, cilantro, mint, lime wedges, and Nuoc Cham dipping sauce.

Nuoc Cham

"Nuoc cham" means "dipping sauce," and this one goes well with the Lemongrass Beef Skewers. This sauce can be made up to 1 day ahead.

MAKES ²/₃ CUP

⅓ cup freshly squeezed lime juice

3 tablespoons fish sauce

1 tablespoon honey

¼ cup water

1 clove garlic, minced

1 Thai bird chili, finely minced, or 1 serrano chili, thinly sliced (feel free to adjust to how much heat you like)

Make the dipping sauce. In a small bowl, combine the lime juice, fish sauce, honey, and water. Mix until honey is dissolved. Add garlic and chili (to taste). Taste for seasoning and adjust to your liking and preferred level of spiciness. The sauce should be salty and slightly funky but balanced by sour and sweetness. Keep covered in the refrigerator until ready to use.

Greens and Herbs Quiche

MAKES 1 (9-INCH) TART
SERVES 6 TO 8

¾ cup finely ground almond flour

¾ cup oat flour

Kosher salt and freshly ground black pepper

3 tablespoons melted refined coconut oil

1 small bunch broccoli rabe, tough ends trimmed (about 2 cups)

1 cup unsweetened almond milk

2 large eggs

1 small shallot, thinly sliced (about 2 tablespoons)

1 clove garlic, peeled and finely chopped

1 cup (lightly packed) chopped mixed herbs, such as parsley, cilantro, dill, and/or chives

½ lemon, zested and cut into wedges, for serving

½ teaspoon ground nutmeg (optional)

When I am craving something creamy and rich but want to skip the dairy, this is my go-to recipe. (And the gluten-free crust can be used in both sweet and savory preparations.)

I love this quiche with broccoli rabe, which has nutty and slightly bitter notes, but the recipe works well with other greens and vegetables like asparagus and mushroom, or blanched broccolini.

When choosing your coconut oil, we recommend using refined coconut oil for this recipe as it has little to no coconut flavor (the unrefined can be a tad too coconutty).

You can store leftovers, cut into wedges, in the freezer for up to a month. To reheat, pop them in a (toaster) oven at 400 degrees for 10 minutes or until heated through.

Make the crust. Preheat the oven to 350 degrees. In a large bowl, combine the almond flour, oat flour, and ½ teaspoon salt. Add the coconut oil and mix thoroughly to combine. The crust mixture will be slightly crumbly but should hold together when squeezed.

Press the crust firmly into a 9-by-1⅛-inch tart pan with a removable bottom, aiming for an equal thickness all around. (You can use your hands, but we've found the flat bottom of a glass or a measuring cup also works.) Prick the bottom and sides of the crust all over with a fork.

Place on a parchment-lined baking sheet and transfer to the oven. Bake until just beginning to turn golden, 13 to 15 minutes. Set aside.

Blanch the greens. Prepare an ice bath. Bring a medium pot of salted water to a rolling boil. Chop the broccoli rabe into ½-inch pieces and blanch in the boiling water, for about 1 minute. You are looking to take the raw edge off but still retain a crunch. Strain and transfer the broccoli rabe immediately to the ice bath to stop the cooking. Drain and squeeze dry.

Prepare the filling. In a large bowl, whisk to combine the almond milk and eggs. Add the broccoli rabe, shallot, garlic, herbs, lemon zest, and nutmeg (if using), and season with ½ teaspoon salt and ¼ teaspoon freshly ground black pepper. Mix well.

Bake. Carefully pour the egg mixture into the quiche crust. Return to the oven and bake until just set, 35 to 45 minutes. (If the crust is browning too fast, tent the whole quiche with foil to prevent overbrowning.)

Let rest. Remove from the oven and let the quiche set for at least 15 minutes. Serve the quiche warm or at room temperature, with lemon wedges on the side.

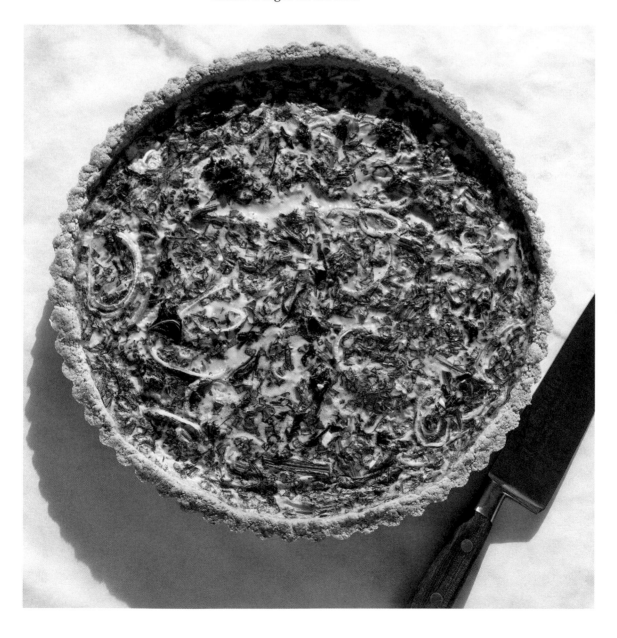

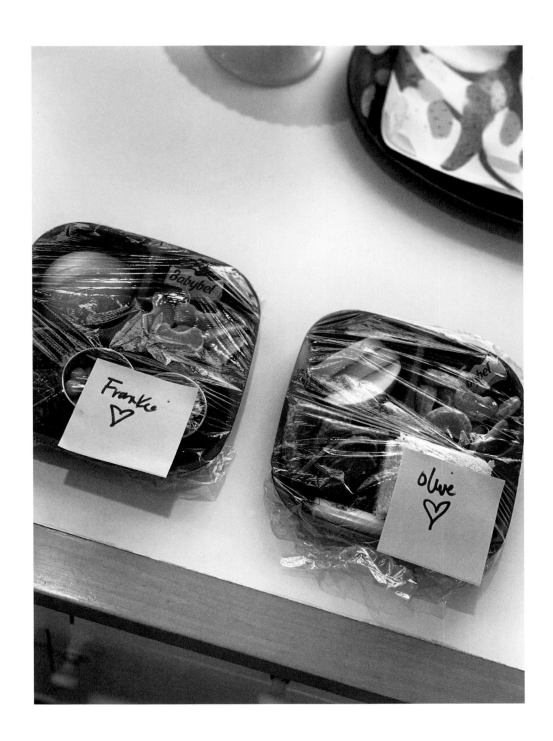

Lather, Rinse, Repeat

One thing I am not is fancy with my kids and food. Frankie has more of an adventurous palate, but Olive kind of likes what she likes. We do a lot of road trips, where they get to eat at their favorite place: the gas station. We get chips and snacks. We allow three treats for each of us—they get something salty and something sweet. We comb the aisles of the gas station marts, and those are moments we treasure as much as a Thanksgiving meal.

As a parent who has had to feed two girls for nine years now, it's been such an odyssey. I've learned to cook steak and salmon and vegetables for them. They love pasta. They love chicken. Then they get in these food ruts when they just don't want to eat anything. Then they only like a certain thing for a while. Then they start to like something new and you're so excited to add it to the repertoire, only to find out the next day that they hate it. And it's really tricky to be a chef for kids. You want to give them healthy food and be responsible, but you're also in parental survival mode, just trying to get through the days and get meals into them, only

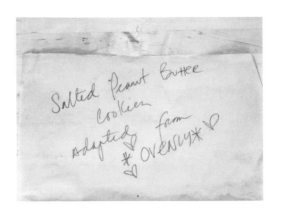

1 3/4 c light brown sugar
2 eggs

*PREHEAT oven to 350°

① WHISK TOGETHER
until completely
crumbled

Then ADD:
1/2 t vanilla
+ whole jar of peanut butter (16.3 oz)
③ whisk until _fully_ incorporated
④ freeze for 15 minutes
⑤ scoop out onto sheet pan w. 2" apart
⑥ freeze for 15 minute
⑦ sprinkle w. sea salt
⑧ BAKE for 15-17 minutes until golden at edges

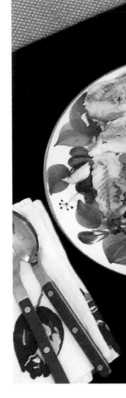

Salted Peanut Butter
Cookies

Adapted from
#OVENLY♥♡

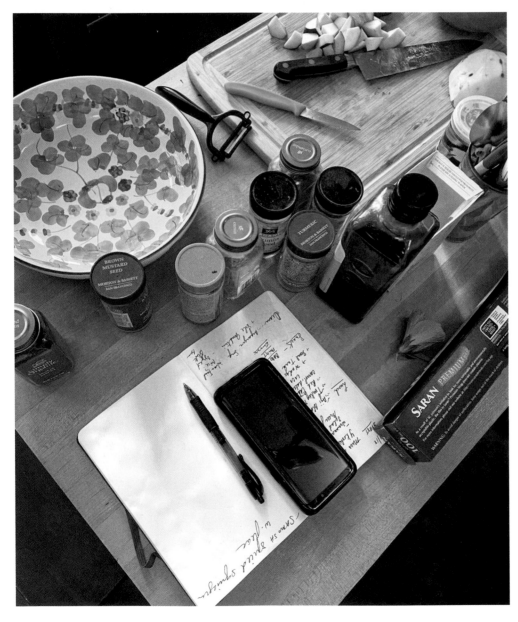

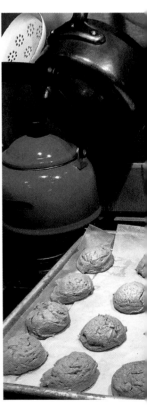

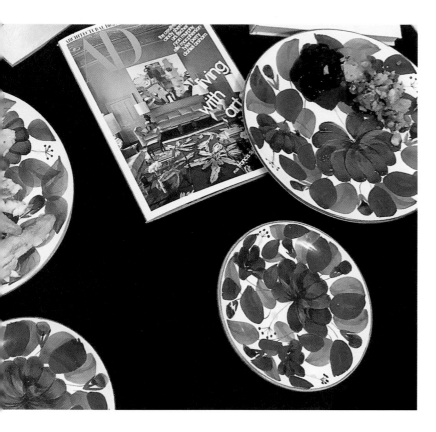

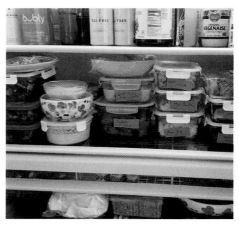

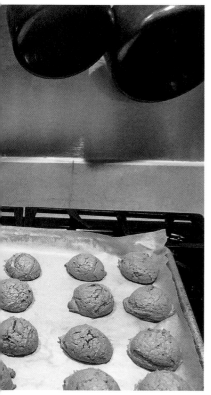

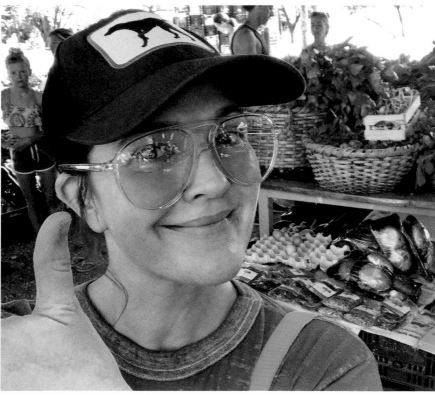

And some days I fail, and some days I feel like I succeed.

to realize that you're letting them snack too much and it's ruining their meals.

It's an ongoing process to be the person who is the food provider for kids as they grow up. That's a whole adventure in food unto itself. But when your kids start learning how to cook popcorn, or surprise you with eggs in the morning, when you finally get a pancake that's on point, it's the greatest. It is so fun for me to cook with my kids, and I've always been messy about it. The flour all over the floor of the kitchen as we bake . . . we've tried to get more responsible and less messy, because those messes can be epic cleanups.

I also don't sit at a table like a Norman Rockwell painting with my kids. We're in the kitchen at a tiny little island in the morning, eating cereal and hard-boiled eggs, getting ready for school. At night, I try to get them to sit at the table, but sometimes they just want to sit on the couch with little tables in front of the TV, and I love that, too. As a parent, you beat up on yourself that the way you do it isn't the right way. But there is no right way. You try to survive and get through the day. And you do your very best. But my food journey since becoming a mom has been not patronizing or overly aspirational. I'm just another parent trying to feed my kids and do the best I can. And some days I fail, and some days I feel like I succeed.

Lather, rinse, repeat.

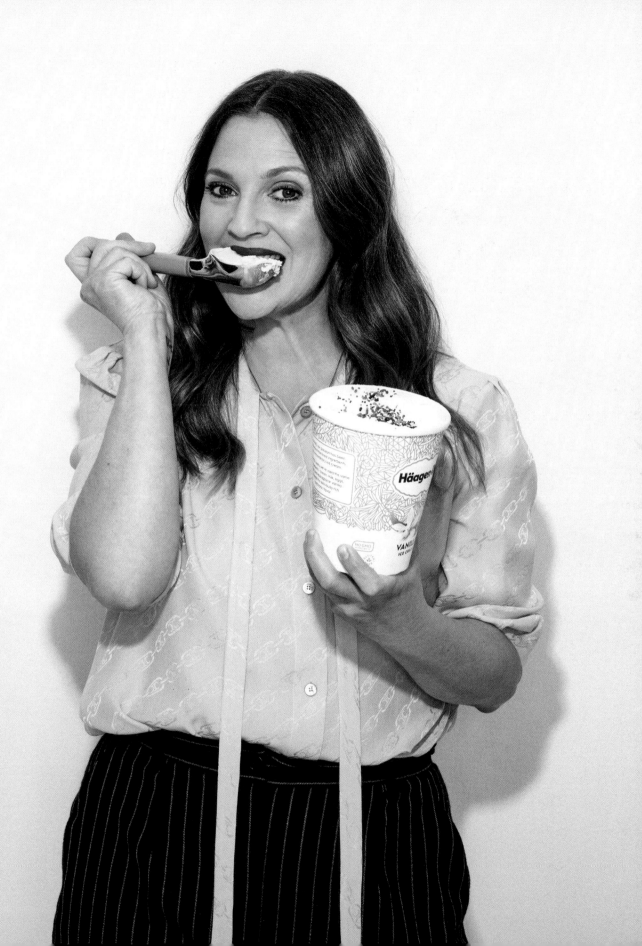

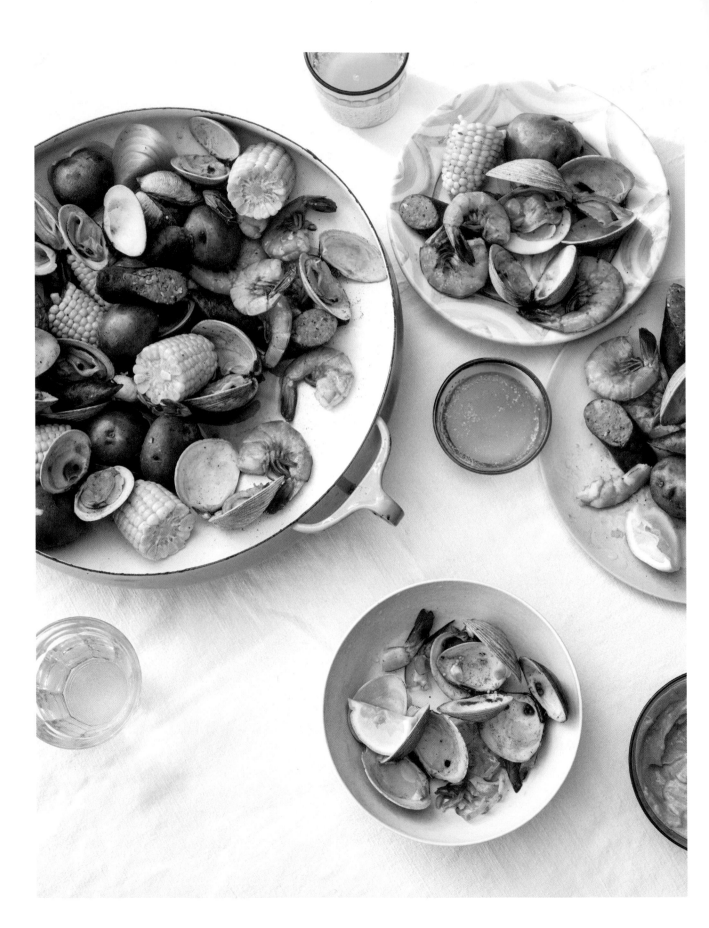

Classic Tradish Seafood Boil

SERVES 4 TO 6

For the Garlic Butter

12 tablespoons (1½ sticks)
   unsalted butter

2 cloves garlic, grated

Kosher salt

*For the Spicy
Mayonnaise*

½ cup mayonnaise
   of choice

Zest of 2 lemons, plus ⅓ cup
   freshly squeezed lemon
   juice

1 small clove garlic, peeled
   and finely grated

1 teaspoon dijon mustard

1½ teaspoon cayenne

Kosher salt and freshly
   ground black pepper

For the Boil

2 lemons, halved, plus
   additional lemon wedges
   for serving

1 orange, halved

1 large yellow onion,
   quartered

5 cloves garlic, smashed

½ small bunch parsley, tied
   with kitchen twine, plus
   more for serving

3 dried bay leaves

(ingredients continue)

Pilar and I are big fans of eating with our hands, and we love a good seafood boil for that reason. There is very minimal prep to this super festive meal—and it has some of our favorite things: *Shrimp! Sausage! Potatoes! Clams! Corn!*

The key to a good seafood boil is making sure that the cooking liquid is full of flavor and placing the ingredients in the pot according to how long they cook—the end result is an incredibly delicious and perfectly cooked boil.

Pull up a chair, roll up your sleeves, and dig in!

Make the garlic butter. Melt the butter in a small pot over medium heat. Using a slotted spoon, skim any foam that comes to the top and discard. Add the garlic, stir to combine, and remove from the heat. Season to taste with salt. (The garlic butter can be made 5 days ahead, stored in an airtight container in the refrigerator.) Rewarm before serving.

Make the spicy mayonnaise. In a small bowl, combine the mayonnaise, lemon zest and juice, garlic, dijon, cayenne, and salt and pepper to taste. (The spicy mayo can be made 5 days ahead, stored in an airtight container in the refrigerator.) Set aside until serving.

Boil. Nestle a steamer basket or steaming insert into a large pot with a tight-fitting lid. (If you don't have a steamer or an insert, prepare a large colander on the side.) Squeeze the lemons and orange into the pot and add the squeezed fruit, along with the onion, garlic, parsley, bay leaves, Old Bay, cayenne, coriander, peppercorns, and 3 tablespoons salt. Add the water. Bring to a boil over high heat and stir to ensure all the salt has dissolved and the flavors infuse, about 10 minutes.

Maintaining a gentle boil, begin to add the components of the boil in increments, based on cooking time. Start with the potatoes: add to the pot, cover and cook for 5 minutes. Next, add the corn and the andouille sausage. After 5 minutes, add the clams and cover. When the clams begin to open up, after about 4 minutes, add the shrimp.

⅓ cup Old Bay

1 tablespoon cayenne

1 tablespoon coriander seeds or pickling spice

1 tablespoon black peppercorns

Kosher salt

18 cups water

1½ pounds small (2-inch) Yukon gold or red bliss potatoes

4 ears corn, shucked and cut into thirds

4 links (12 ounces) andouille sausage, sliced crosswise into 1½-inch pieces

24 littleneck clams, rinsed well

1½ pounds (16/20) shell-on shrimp, backs split and inner tract removed

Using tongs, nestle the shrimp into the cooking liquid and cover the pot. Continue cooking for 1 minute. Turn the heat off, leaving the lid on, and let the boil sit until the shrimp is cooked through and all clams have opened, 2 to 4 minutes more.

Remove the lid and carefully lift the steamer basket out of the water. (If not using an insert, gently drain the contents of the pot into a large colander.) Discard the liquid.

Serve. Place the boil ingredients on a large serving platter (or on some newspaper!) and serve with the garlic butter, spicy mayonnaise, and lemon wedges on the side. Enjoy while steaming hot.

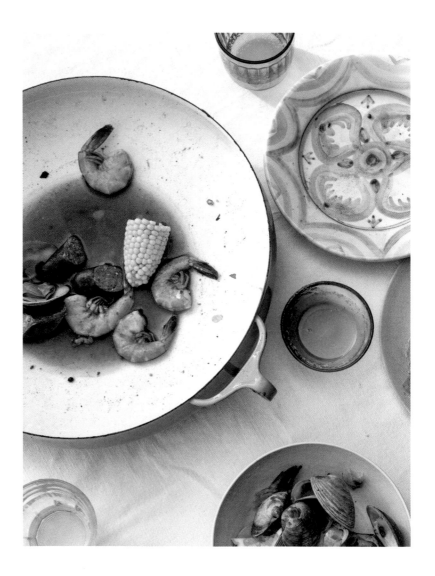

1 to 1¼ pounds winter squash (recommend delicata, butternut, or acorn squash)

Kosher salt and freshly ground black pepper

2 tablespoons avocado oil, divided

2½ cups Homemade Vegetable Stock (see page 54) or water, separated

1 cup white quinoa

4 ounces king trumpet mushrooms (or 2 cups sliced mushrooms of your choice), bases trimmed, cut lengthwise into ¼-inch slices and scored

1 scallion, green and white parts, thinly sliced crosswise

Leaves from 2 sprigs parsley

1 lemon, zested and cut into wedges for serving

Autumn Hug in a Bowl (Quinoa Risotto with Squash, Herbs, and Seared Mushrooms)

This dish was the first thing Pilar and I made together on the show, and it's exactly what it sounds like—warm, cozy, and comforting! It is basically a quinoa risotto with a yummy squash puree standing in for the more traditional cream, making it 100 percent vegan.

Roast the squash. Preheat the oven to 400 degrees. Halve the squash, scoop out the seeds (save for another use), and cut into half-moon slices, ½ inch thick. Season lightly with salt and pepper and drizzle with 2 teaspoons avocado oil. Roast until tender and golden, 20 to 25 minutes. Allow to cool slightly. Place 1 cup of cooked squash and ¼ cup Homemade Vegetable Stock in a blender and blend until smooth. Season to taste.

Cook the quinoa. Place a medium pot over medium heat. Add the quinoa and toast, stirring frequently, until the quinoa is fragrant and a hue darker, about 2 minutes. Remove the pot from the heat and very slowly pour in the remaining 2¼ cups Homemade Vegetable Stock, being very careful as it will spatter. Season with a pinch of salt and pepper. Return to the heat, adjusting to maintain a brisk simmer, and cook, stirring occasionally, until cooked through, about 18 minutes. It should be looser than regular cooked quinoa, but each seed should still have some shape. Fold in the squash puree. Check the seasoning and adjust as necessary.

Sear the mushrooms. Heat a skillet over medium-high heat. Add 1 tablespoon avocado oil and swirl to coat. Sear the mushrooms on each side until golden brown and just cooked through, 2 to 3 minutes per side. Remove from the heat. Season the mushrooms with salt and pepper.

Serve. Place the warm, creamy quinoa in bowls. Top with remaining squash and seared mushrooms. Garnish with scallion and parsley leaves, lemon zest, and a squeeze of lemon. Drizzle the remaining avocado oil on top and finish with freshly ground black pepper.

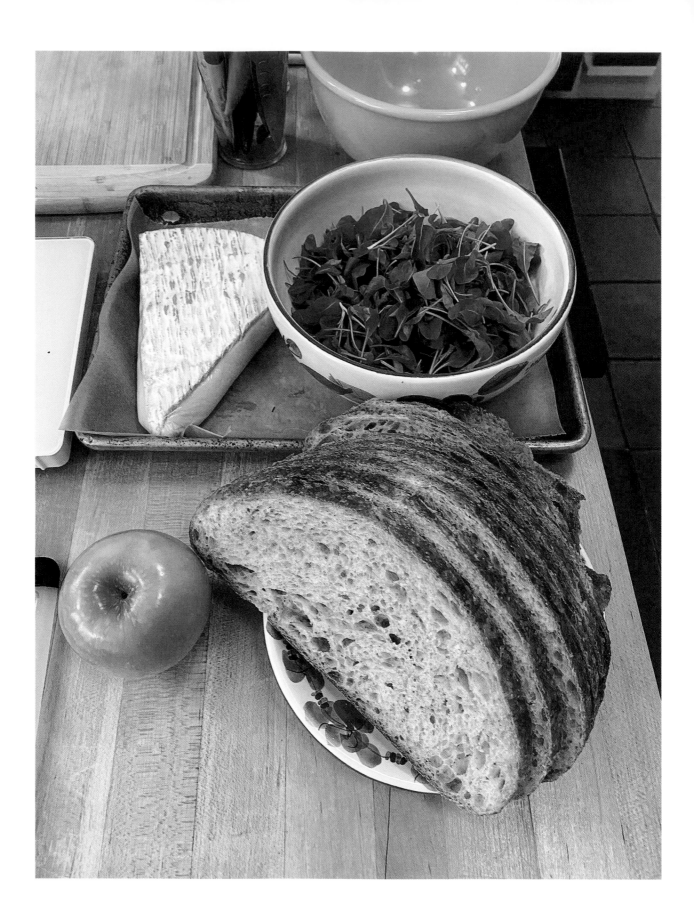

Brie and Apple Grilled Cheese

MAKES 1 SANDWICH

2 pieces sourdough bread, cut into ½-inch-thick slices

1½ tablespoons unsalted butter, at room temperature, divided

2 teaspoons Colman's prepared mustard, plus additional for serving

6 thin slices Granny Smith apple

2½ ounces Brie, slightly chilled

1 large handful arugula (about 1 cup)

I love this recipe because I love loading up on cheese and carbs some days, but I still want peppery arugula and sweet, crisp, tart apple in the mix, too. I guess I'm saying I want it all, and I really, truly believe this sandwich has it! I learned to make it when I was eight months pregnant and in a Los Angeles August heat wave. And that still didn't stop me from wanting a gooey, yummy, multi-textured sandwich that lives on in my heart.

I believe the key to success is to pre-butter the bread before it hits the pan. I cannot stress this enough! Another pro tip is to put the arugula on top of the brie, as it acts as a perfect culinary adhesive.

Butter the bread. Slather one side of each slice of bread with ½ tablespoon butter. Place the bread slices buttered-side down on a work surface.

Assemble the sandwich. Spread mustard on one side. On the opposite side, shingle the apple slices.

Remove the rind from the Brie and discard (or eat!). Lay the Brie on top of the apple, spreading and flattening as much as possible. Add arugula and press to adhere. Close with the other piece of bread so that both buttered sides are on the outside.

Cook. Heat a skillet over medium heat. Add ½ tablespoon butter and swirl to coat. When sizzling, add the sandwich, and press down with a spatula to encourage even toasting. Cook until golden and crispy, 2 to 3 minutes, adjusting the heat as necessary to prevent burning. Flip the sandwich. Continue cooking, lightly pressing with a spatula, until the bread is golden and the cheese is melty, about 2 minutes more.

Serve. Transfer to a cutting board and cut in half. Serve immediately, with additional mustard on the side.

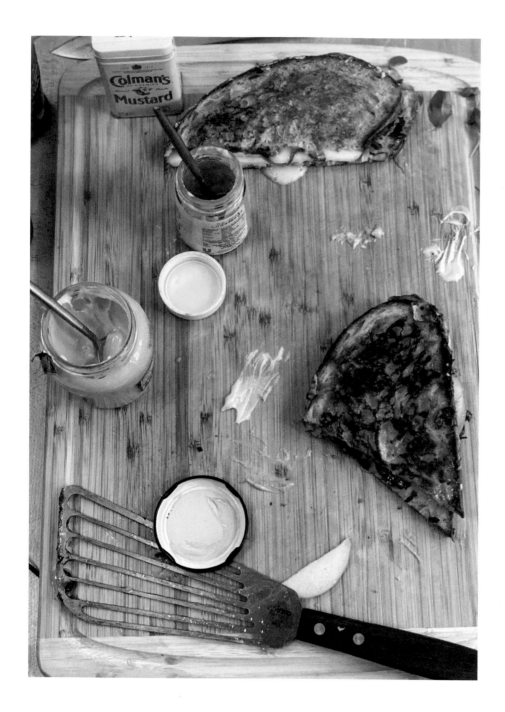

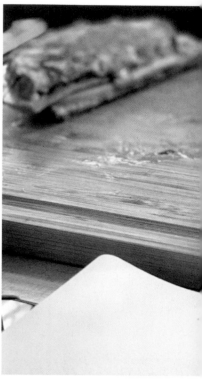

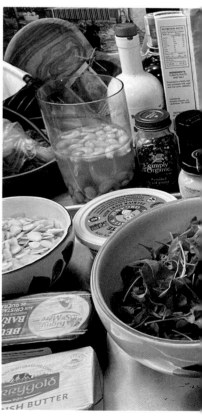

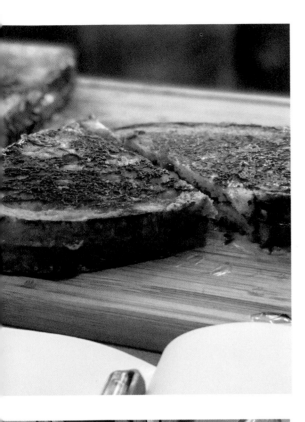

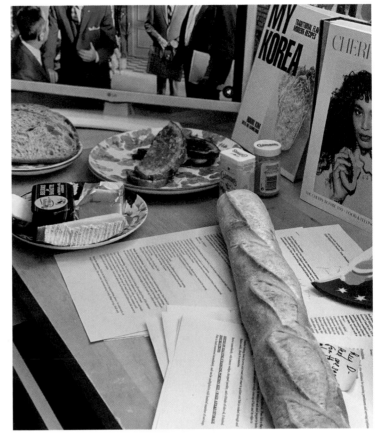

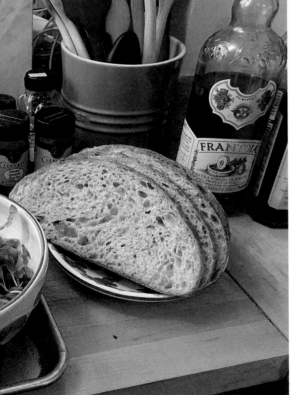

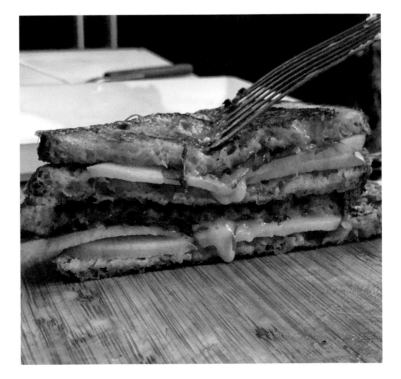

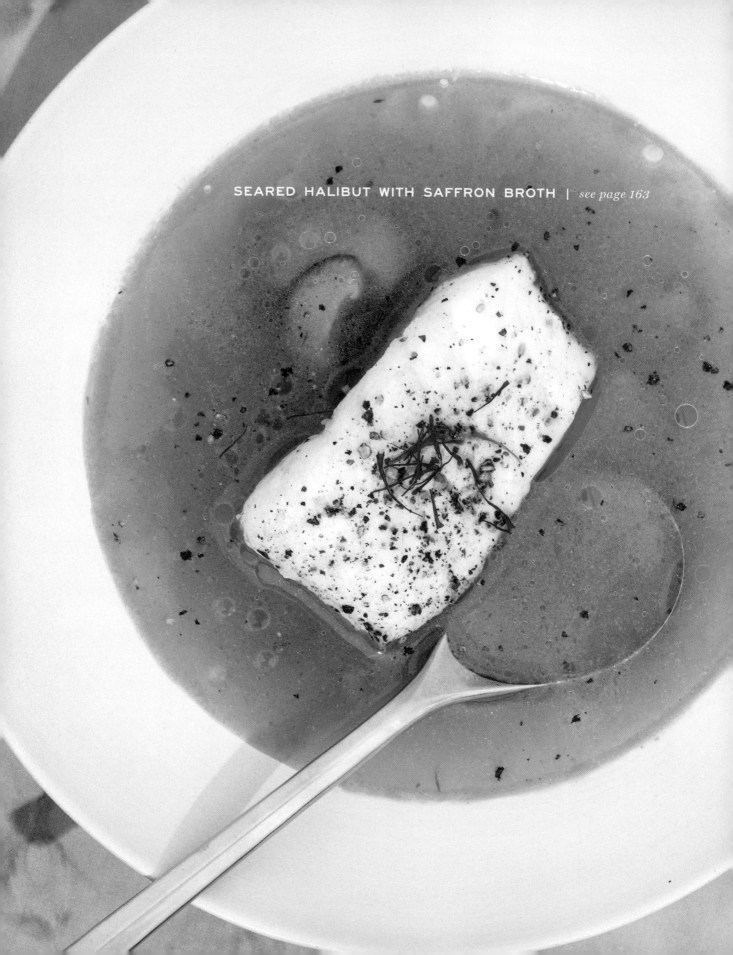

SEARED HALIBUT WITH SAFFRON BROTH | *see page 163*

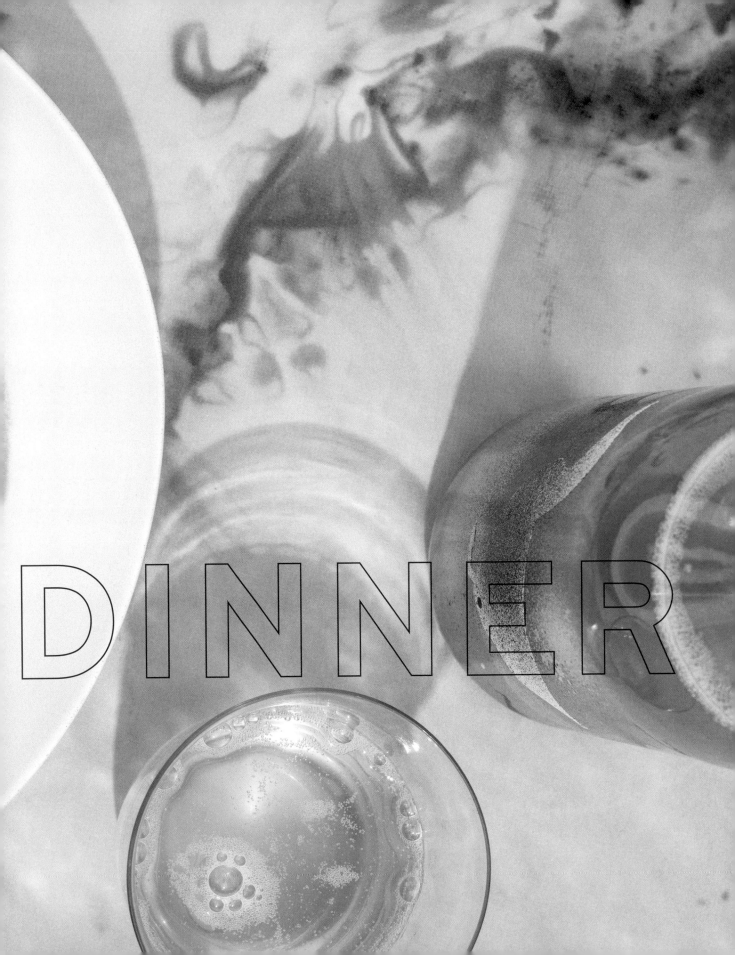

DINNER

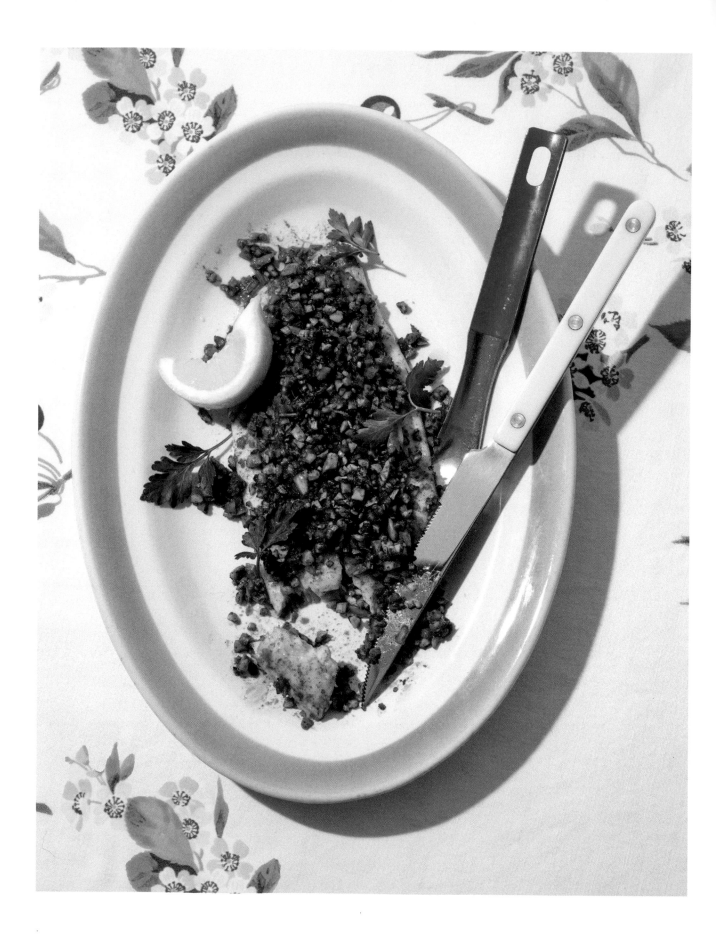

Nutty Fish

SERVES 1

¼ cup blanched, slivered
   almonds

¼ teaspoon ground cumin

¼ teaspoon pimenton
   (aka smoked paprika)

2 tablespoons minced shallot
   (1 medium shallot)

2 tablespoons minced parsley
   stems, leaves reserved for
   garnish

1 lemon, zested and cut into
   wedges

Kosher salt and freshly
   ground black pepper

3 teaspoons olive oil, divided

1 skinless fillet of delicate
   white fish, such as sole,
   fluke, or flounder (about
   6 to 8 ounces)

Cooking and eating for one is not always the most fun (or inspiring), and Pilar and I wanted to create a delectable dish that was only *slightly* more involved than tapping away at your favorite delivery app.

Save for the fish, you probably have most of the ingredients on hand already. We love shallots for their delicate sweetness and flavor, but if you can't get your hands on those, red onion would be a nice substitute. When chopping up the almonds for this recipe, don't worry too much about chopping them all the same size—or too finely. The texture gives a really great crunch and crust that complements the delicate fish nicely.

This recipe can be dispatched in under half an hour—perfect for solo date-night vibes.

Toast the nuts. Preheat oven to 350 degrees. Line a small sheet pan with parchment paper. Place the almonds in a single layer on the sheet pan, and toast them in the oven until slightly golden and fragrant, 8 to 10 minutes, shaking the pan halfway through. Allow them to cool, then roughly chop. Variation in texture and size is what we are looking for—but nothing larger than a pea.

Raise your oven temperature to 375 degrees.

Make the crust. Transfer your roughly chopped almonds to a medium bowl. Add the cumin, smoked paprika, shallot, parsley stems, 1 teaspoon lemon zest, and a pinch of salt and black pepper to the bowl and mix until combined. Drizzle 2 teaspoons of olive oil and give it one last stir, until the olive oil is evenly distributed.

Prepare the fish. Pat the fish dry and season both sides with salt and pepper. Using the same sheet pan you used to toast the almonds, drizzle the remaining olive oil on the pan and place the fillet in the center. Spread the almond mixture evenly on top, pressing ever so gently to form a crust. Make sure to cover the fillet end to end.

Roast. Transfer the prepared fish to the oven, using the top rack, and roast until the crust is golden and the fish is cooked through and flakes easily, 8 to 9 minutes.

Serve immediately. Top with parsley leaves and lemon wedges on the side. We think it goes great with roasted asparagus or Pairs with Everything Salad (page 213).

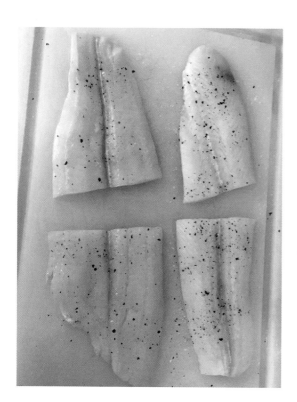
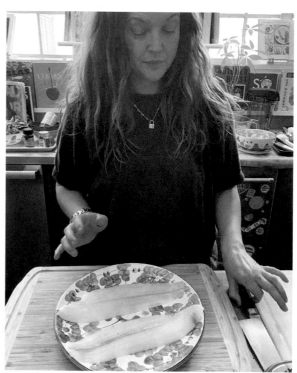

My Favorite Shredded Beef

SERVES 4 TO 6

1½ tablespoons paprika

Kosher salt and freshly ground black pepper

2½ pounds beef chuck, trimmed and cut into 2- to 3-inch cubes

1 heaping tablespoon cumin seeds

1 heaping tablespoon coriander seeds

2 tablespoons avocado oil, plus additional as necessary

1 large onion, peeled and chopped into 1-inch pieces

2 celery stalks, cut crosswise into 2-inch pieces, including leaves

2 medium carrots, peeled and cut crosswise into 2-inch pieces

1 jalapeño, thinly sliced crosswise (and seeded, if preference is for more mild)

2 chipotles in adobo sauce, chopped (optional)

5 cloves garlic, peeled and smashed

1 tablespoon dried Mexican oregano

1 (28-ounce) can San Marzano tomatoes, chopped

3 cups water, plus more if necessary

1 dried bay leaf

(ingredients continue)

I don't eat a lot of meat, but when I do, 90 percent of the time it's probably gonna be in Mexican food. And I have a real weakness for this dish, which is inspired by tinga de res, in all its shredded beef glory. I love heat and spice, but I don't love chipotles in adobo, so when I make this dish I leave them out and load up on more vegetables, which is a departure from the traditional.

A quick note about cutting the beef: the larger the cubes, the longer the shred, so if you like that really stringy texture, the larger cut is for you.

The beef cooks on the stovetop and fills the house with the most glorious aroma; everyone heads to the kitchen to see what's cooking. Make it in advance (it's better the next day). This also freezes and reheats really nicely.

Make the rub. In a small bowl, combine the paprika, 1½ tablespoons salt, and 2 teaspoons freshly ground black pepper.

Make the beef. Sprinkle beef with the spice mixture on all sides to fully coat it. (The beef can be seasoned with the spice mixture up to 2 days in advance. Keep covered, in the refrigerator, until ready to cook.)

Place the cumin and coriander seeds in a small skillet over medium-high heat. Toast, shaking the skillet occasionally, until the spices are fragrant and just beginning to smoke, 1 to 2 minutes.

Heat a large heavy-bottomed pot (like a Dutch oven) over medium-high heat. Add the avocado oil and swirl to coat. When shimmering, add the beef and sear until deeply golden, about 3 minutes per side, reducing the heat as necessary to prevent the spices from burning. Remove the beef to a plate and add an additional 1 tablespoon avocado oil if the pan looks dry. (This will depend on how lean the beef is.)

Add the onions, celery, carrots, jalapeño, chipotles (if using), and garlic, season with salt and pepper, and cook, stirring occasionally, until softened and lightly caramelized, 8 to 10 minutes. Add the coriander, cumin, and Mexican oregano and continue cooking until the spices are toasted and fragrant, 1 to 2 minutes. Add the

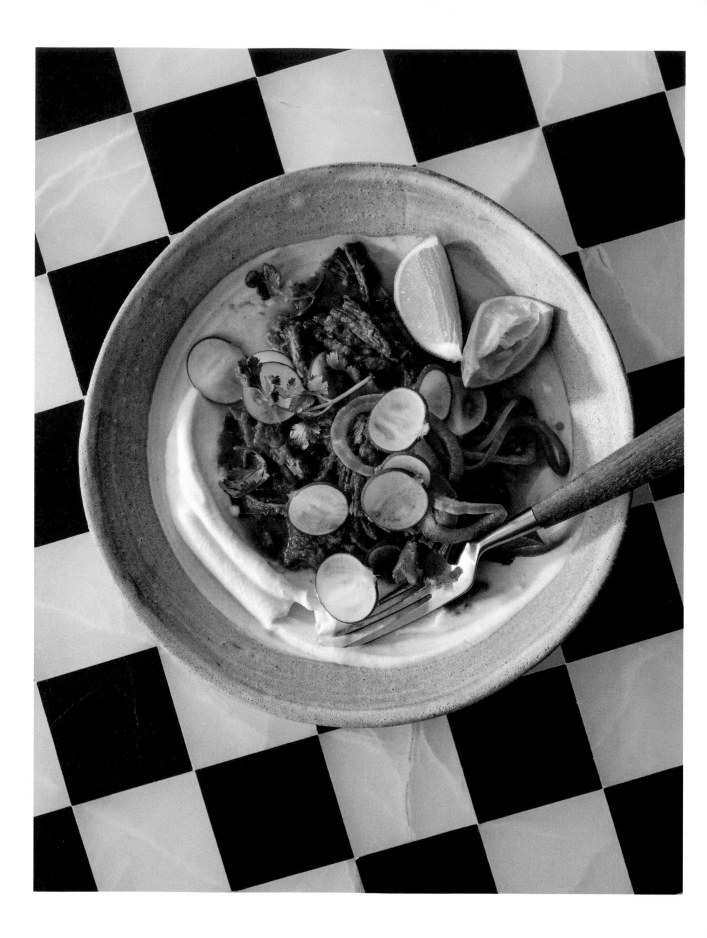

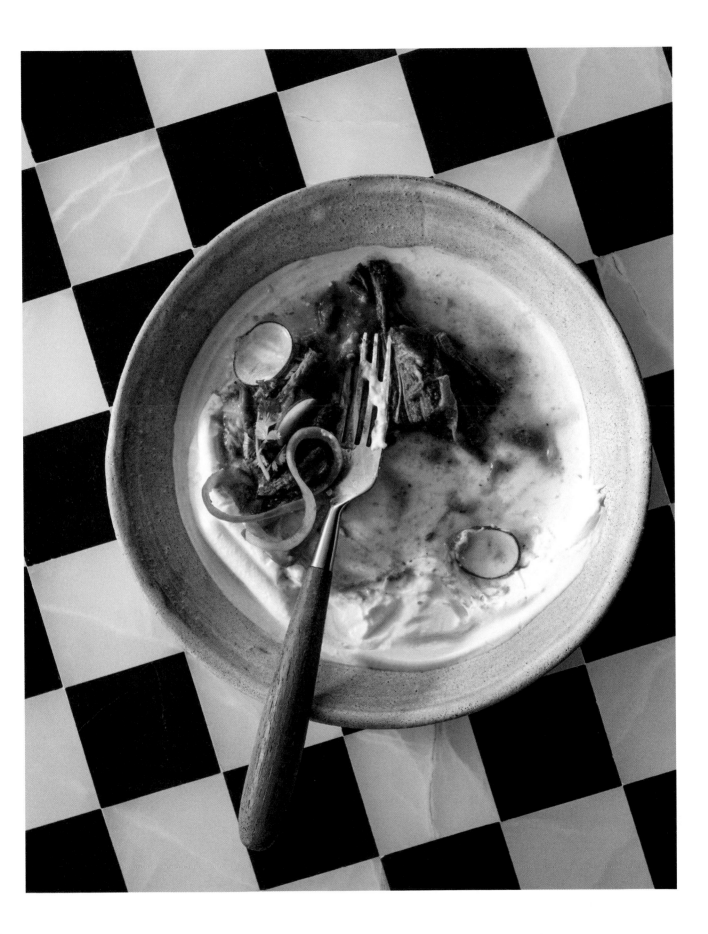

5 cloves

1 bunch cilantro, leaves
reserved, stems tied
together with kitchen twine

For Serving

**Quick-Pickled Red Onions
(recipe follows)**

Cilantro

Lime wedges

Thinly sliced radishes

Your favorite tortillas

Mexican oregano

Coconut yogurt (optional)

tomatoes, water, bay leaf, cloves, and cilantro stems, scraping the bottom of the pot to deglaze. Nestle the beef pieces into the pot, including any accumulated juices from the plate. The liquid level should come just to the top of the meat. Add water to adjust, if necessary. Bring to a boil and cover the pot, with the lid slightly ajar. Reduce the heat to maintain a brisk simmer and braise, basting the top of the meat with sauce every 30 minutes, until the beef easily shreds with a fork, 2½ to 3 hours.

Finish the sauce. Remove the cilantro bundle. Transfer the beef to a plate and keep covered. Carefully transfer the contents of the pot to a blender, reserving about 1 cup of the vegetables, and blend until the mixture is very smooth. If necessary, add water, 1 tablespoon at a time, to reach a thick yet pourable consistency. Season to taste with salt and pepper.

Shred the beef with two forks and return to the pot, along with the reserved 1 cup of vegetables and the blended sauce. Stir to combine and keep warm until ready to serve.

Serve. Divide the beef and sauce among shallow serving bowls and serve, topped with pickled red onions, a spoonful of pickling aromatics, reserved cilantro leaves, lime wedges, radishes, tortillas, Mexican oregano, and coconut yogurt, if desired.

Quick-Pickled Red Onions

1 medium red onion, peeled and thinly sliced crosswise into rings

½ cup red wine vinegar

1 cup water

1½ tablespoons sugar

1 tablespoon kosher salt

1 teaspoon cumin seed

1 teaspoon fennel seed

1 teaspoon coriander seed

1 teaspoon black peppercorns

1 bay leaf

Place the onions in a mason jar or medium bowl. In a medium pot, combine the remaining ingredients. Bring to a boil over high heat, stirring to dissolve the sugar and salt. Pour the pickling liquid over the onions, pressing them down to make sure they are completely submerged.

Cover and transfer to the refrigerator. Let sit at least 1 hour before using. These can be prepared up to 5 days in advance.

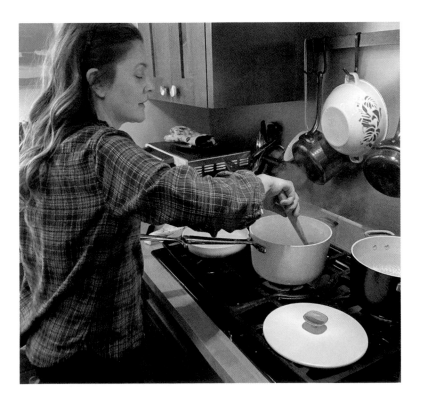

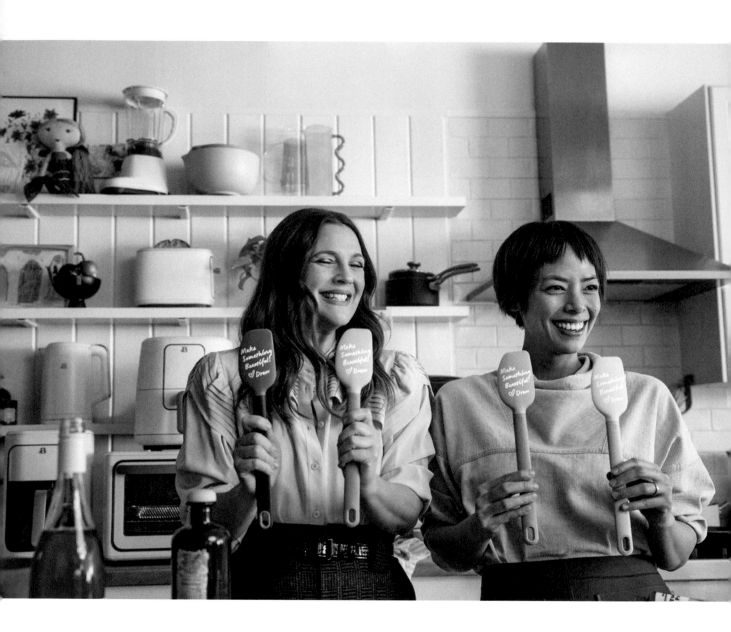

Serve Hot!

Drew: Pilar and I had this very important person to cook for, one of those high-stake meals where we were really trying to impress.

Pilar: It was impressive on so many levels.

Drew: We had set the menu, using a recipe from this book, the Chickpea Carbonara (page 147). Pilar was to make it, and I was to entertain the person. We had planned it for weeks. The morning of, everything was all set. I did the entertaining part, but I did it for too long—like an hour too long. Pilar's food got ice-cold.

Pilar: And rock-hard! Drew is a wonderful, wonderful . . .

Drew: I fucked up my side of things! I over-entertained!

Pilar: I think it was at that point we decided when the food is ready, the food is ready. And this dish, the Chickpea Carbonara, must be eaten hot. And we learned that the very hard way.

Drew: The very hardest way. I felt so bad I had rats in my stomach, and the whole meal took a complete nosedive, engulfed in flames. Pilar's and my goal of impressing this person ended up with some mea culpas, some road bumps with each other. But we came out of it with flying colors.

And to this day, Chickpea Carbonara will remind us of an important moment gone horribly wrong.

Pilar: It's okay. A learning moment. We're better for it. We survived out of the ashes!

Drew: And this dish, more than any other, we will always say, SERVE HOT.

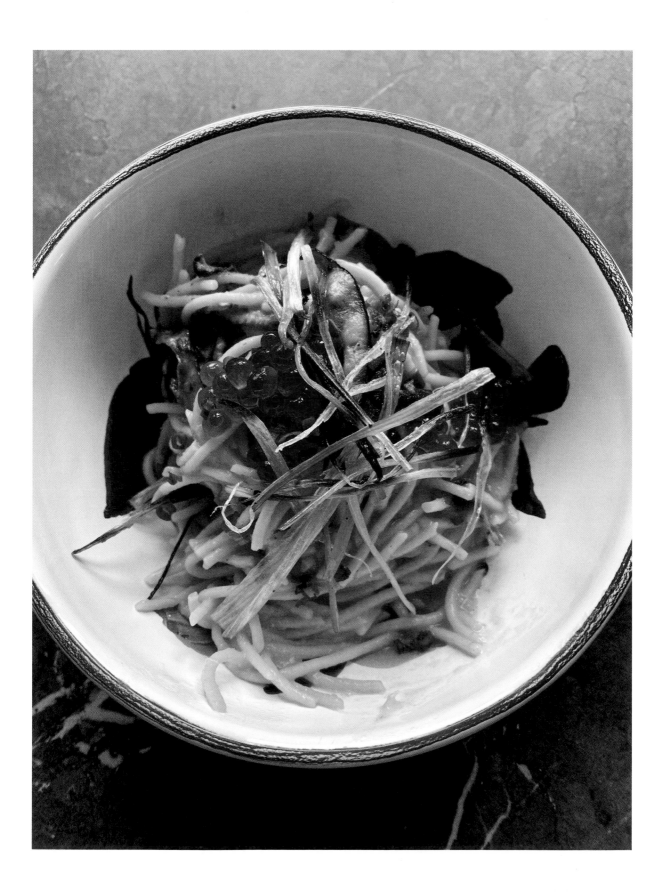

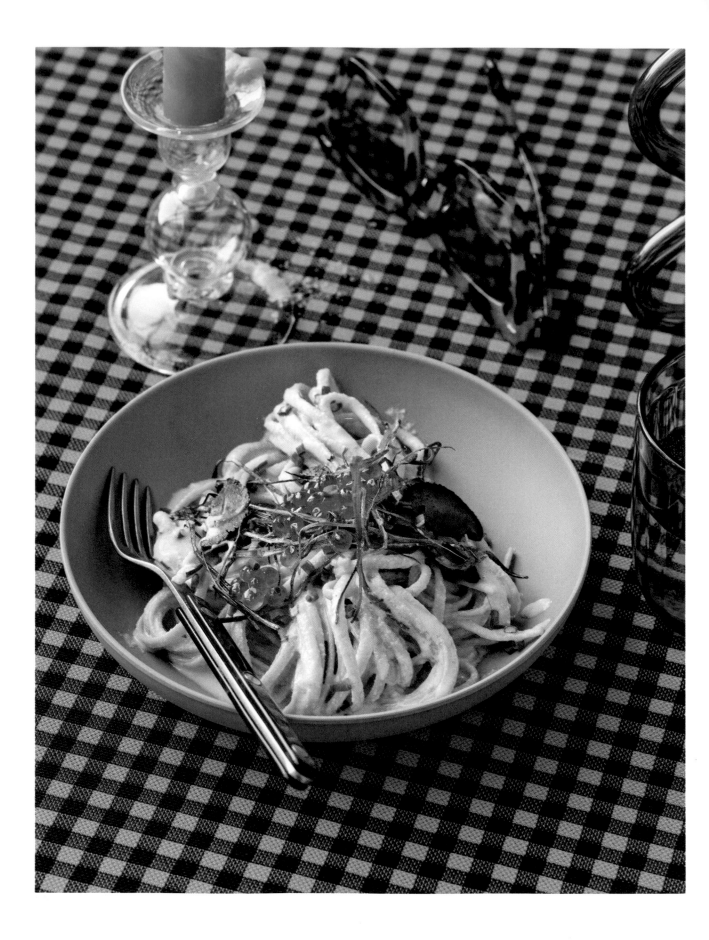

Chickpea Carbonara with Shiitake Bacon and Crispy Leeks

For Leek-Miso Sauce

2 tablespoons olive oil

2 large leeks, white and light green parts only, thinly cut crosswise (about 2 cups)

Kosher salt and freshly ground black pepper

2 tablespoons water

1 heaping tablespoon chickpea miso paste or white miso paste

½ cup aquafaba (bean-soaking liquid) from 1 (15.5-ounce) can chickpeas (store chickpeas in water for another use)

For Shiitake Bacon and Crispy Leeks

1 large leek, white and light green part only, halved lengthwise and very thinly sliced lengthwise into 3- to 4-inch julienne (about 1 heaping cup)

5 ounces shiitake mushrooms, destemmed and cut into ⅛-inch slices (about 2 heaping cups)

2 tablespoons olive oil

½ teaspoon smoked paprika

Kosher salt and freshly ground black pepper

(ingredients continue)

I love pasta and cheese, but there are definitely times when I feel like I need to cut back a little. Working with Pilar to create these recipes, I wasn't necessarily looking for vegan or gluten-free versions of dishes, but rather dishes that embrace the spirit of some of my favorite things, satisfying and delicious in their own right. I think this recipe really captures that. We like to think of this recipe as a cross between a Japanese mentaiko pasta and an Italian carbonara. It highlights some tips and tricks we use throughout the book—using purees to add creaminess, playing with texture to give dishes a crunch and craveability, loading up on acid to keep things bright and light. (You can also keep the roe off to make the dish vegan.) And the shiitake and leek garnish is ridiculously addictive. Try not to snack on them all before garnishing the dish!

Preheat the oven to 375 degrees.

Make the leek-miso sauce. Heat olive oil in a large skillet over medium heat. Add the sliced leeks, season with salt and pepper, and sauté, stirring occasionally, until the leeks are softened and begin to turn lightly golden, 10 to 12 minutes. Adjust the heat as necessary to prevent burning. Add the water and stir, scraping the bottom of the pan to deglaze. Transfer the mixture to a blender. Add the miso paste and the aquafaba and blend until completely smooth. Season to taste with salt.

Make the shiitake bacon and crispy leeks. Place the julienned leeks and sliced shiitake mushrooms on a rimmed sheet pan and drizzle with olive oil. Season with smoked paprika, salt, and pepper and toss to coat. Spread the vegetables out in a single layer. Roast, stirring twice during cooking, until the leeks and shiitakes are crisped and golden, 20 to 25 minutes. Remove from the oven and let cool.

Finish the pasta. Bring a large pot of salted water to a boil over high heat. Add the chickpea linguini and cook according to the

1 (8-ounce) package chickpea linguini (we recommend Banza)

¼ cup finely chopped chives, divided

1 teaspoon yuzu juice (or 1 teaspoon freshly squeezed lime juice)

2 to 3 tablespoons fish roe, like salmon or trout, for serving (optional)

package instructions, stirring occasionally, until just tender, about 6 minutes. Do not overcook. Reserve 1 cup of pasta water and set aside. Drain the noodles and rinse thoroughly with cold water to stop the cooking.

Reduce the heat to medium low and return the pasta to the pot and add the leek-miso sauce, ½ cup of pasta water, and 2 tablespoons of chives. Toss to combine. Continue thinning the sauce with up to ½ cup more pasta water if needed, folding gently to combine with the noodles, until the sauce is velvety and the pasta is very generously coated. The noodles should feel *nearly* overdressed, as the pasta will continue absorbing the sauce as it sits.

Serve. Add the yuzu juice, plenty of black pepper, and season with salt to taste. Divide among serving bowls, and top with remaining 2 tablespoons chives, shiitake bacon, crispy leeks, and roe (if using). Serve Hot!

Ode to Campbell's Cream of Mushroom Soup

MAKES 5 CUPS
SERVES 4

10 ounces cremini mushrooms, stems removed and reserved, sliced (about 4 cups)

5 ounces shiitake mushrooms, stems removed and reserved, sliced (2 heaping cups)

1½ cups roughly chopped cauliflower, trimmings, ends, outer leaves, and core reserved

2 stalks celery, roughly chopped (about 1 scant cup), trimmings and ends reserved

½ teaspoon whole black peppercorns

4 sprigs thyme

1 bay leaf

1 tablespoon olive oil

1 small clove garlic, minced

Kosher salt and freshly ground black pepper

½ cup plain, unsweetened almond milk

½ teaspoon tamari (or soy sauce if not keeping gluten-free), plus additional if desired, for seasoning

½ teaspoon balsamic vinegar, plus additional if desired, for seasoning

1 tablespoon chives, finely chopped, for garnish

This iconic red-and-white can is something that is very personal for Pilar and me. As we were getting to know each other and becoming friends, we discovered that both of our moms made our favorite childhood dishes with none other than the same ingredient . . . Campbell's Cream of Mushroom Soup. For me it was my mom's tuna noodle casserole; I think it's my first food memory. And for Pilar, when she was growing up in Manila and would get a cold, her mom would treat her to a hot bowl of Campbell's Cream of Mushroom Soup. So we decided to put our two hearts into one bowl and create our own new adult version of the classic. We hope you enjoy.

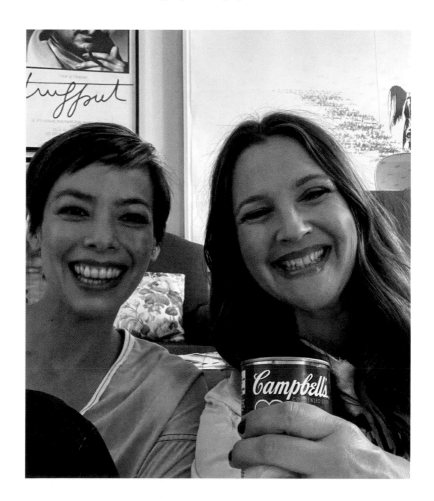

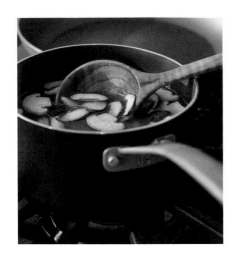

Make the mushroom stock. Fill a medium pot with 6 cups of water. Add the mushroom stems, cauliflower trimmings, celery trimmings, black peppercorns, thyme, and bay leaf. Place over high heat and bring to a boil, adjusting the heat as necessary to maintain a brisk simmer, for 10 to 20 minutes. Remove from the heat, strain through a fine-mesh strainer, and discard the solids. (Mushroom stock can be made up to 3 days in advance and kept in an airtight container in the refrigerator, or frozen for up to 3 months.)

Make the soup. Meanwhile, heat a large pot over medium-high heat. Add the olive oil. When shimmering, add the celery and garlic, season with salt and pepper, and sauté for 1½ to 2 minutes, until the celery begins to turn translucent and the garlic is fragrant. Reduce the heat if necessary to prevent browning. Add cauliflower florets and season with salt and pepper. Cook, stirring occasionally, until the cauliflower is slightly softened but still has a bite, about 2 minutes. Taste as you go—not just for seasoning but for texture as well. Add the cremini and shiitake mushrooms. Continue sautéing until the mushrooms begin to release liquid and brown, 3 to 4 minutes.

Remove ½ cup of the mushroom mixture and set aside. Add 4 cups of the strained mushroom stock to the mushroom mixture in the pot, along with the almond milk, tamari, balsamic vinegar, and a dash of black pepper. Bring to a boil and then reduce to a simmer.

Blend. Continue to simmer for 10 more minutes, until the flavors marry and the liquid is slightly reduced. Transfer the contents of the pot to a blender and blend until smooth. Taste for seasoning and adjust with more salt, pepper, tamari, and/or balsamic vinegar.

Serve. Divide the reserved mushroom mixture into serving bowls and ladle the hot soup on top. Garnish with freshly ground black pepper and chives.

Thanksgiving

Drew: I remember the first Thanksgiving we had in our house, the one I bought after moving from the West Coast. I moved in October, just in time for a first Thanksgiving, and Pilar created this beautiful menu and did a drawing and an illustration. We made it a really festive occasion. Pilar, what are your memories from that day?

Pilar: I remember getting there fairly early in the morning since we were eating at around 1:00 or 1:30. I think I got there at 4:30 in the morning. It was still dark out. I was really trying not to wake anyone up, but of course I was in my freaking clunky-ass boots! So I think I pretty much woke up Drew and Frankie—I'm so sorry, guys; don't mind me! I have a nine-hundred-pound turkey!

There were so many moments from that day that were special. I remember your table that looked like it was only going to seat four, but it magically expanded.

Drew: We had this magical table that could seat up to fifteen.

Pilar: It really was magical! It just kept giving and giving.

Drew: I bought it at ABC Carpet and Home because I had never seen a table like that. It's a Danish design. It folds up into a small console table, and it expands to a table that can easily seat twelve. But I think we had fifteen or twenty people there, all friends and family, right before the pandemic.

Pilar: Five months before. I think that was the first gathering we had in the house to really get it properly warmed. We still had the old oven in, and I was really bracing to see if it could handle the turkey.

Drew: We did an ode to our love of Campbell's Cream of Mushroom Soup, our connector, with a green bean casserole.

Pilar: We went with a fairly traditional menu, which was exciting to me. I had never made a green bean casserole, and I'd never had it, because I didn't grow up in the United States. There's folklore about it; you hear about it all the time. But I hadn't made it before. You needed some sort of cream of mushroom soup, and I love Campbell's, so I made my own ode to Campbell's Cream of Mushroom Soup from scratch. The recipe is in the book (page 149). It's a cauliflower base with lots of mushrooms.

Drew: And it doesn't taste cauliflowery.

Pilar: It's really light. You use a ton of mushrooms, and then you get it really nice and creamy. And then you top it with a lot of French's fried onions.

Drew: You can't replace those. They know what they're doing.

Pilar: Classic for a reason!

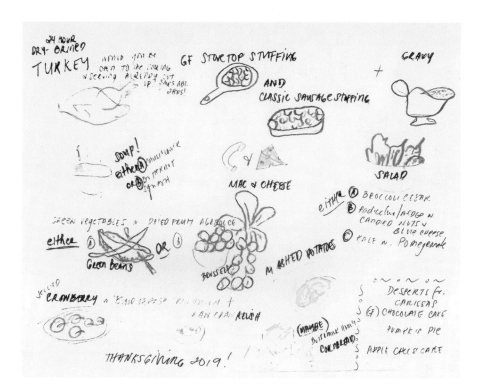

Drew: Our friends were all there and made it so much fun! Chris sent a piñata, and all the kids hit it outside. And you and I and Gabe took pictures with our old cameras, then we developed the film.

Pilar: It was such a happy day. It wasn't too cold, so we were outside, slightly bundled, in the sun and the light.

Drew: It was a perfect Thanksgiving, a drop-the-mic Thanksgiving.

   I don't even remember what this last Thanksgiving was in the pandemic. I don't remember it at all.

Pilar: Me neither!

Drew: Get ready, Thanksgiving 2021, we're coming for you!

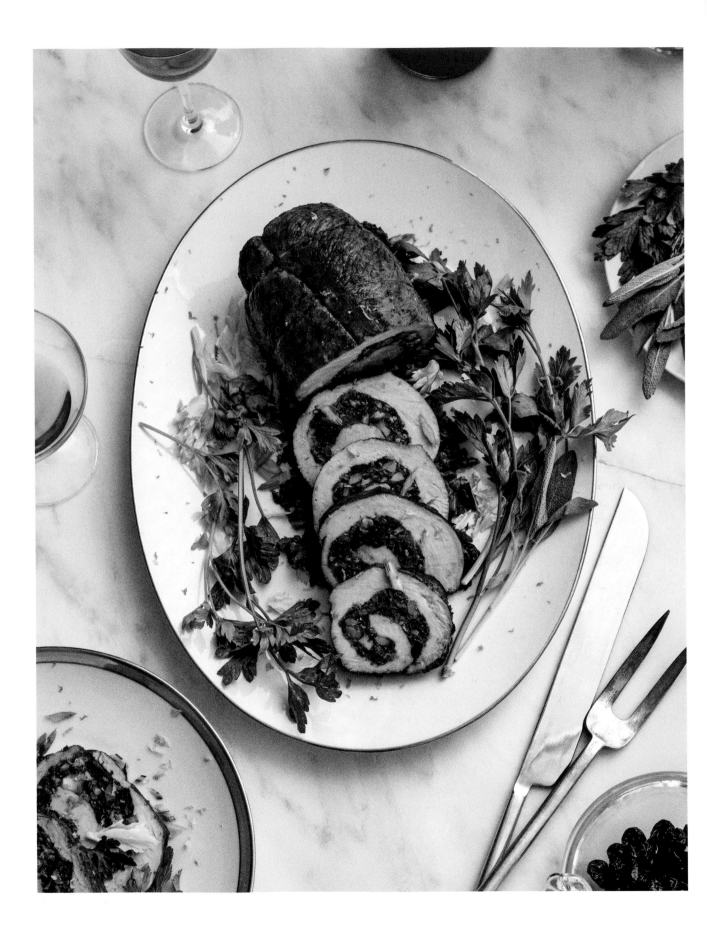

Thanksgiving Roulade

SERVES 4 TO 6, WITH
LEFTOVERS

For the Roulade

2½ teaspoons granulated
   sugar

Kosher salt and freshly
   ground black pepper

2 pounds boneless, skinless
   turkey breast, butterflied
   and pounded to ½ inch
   thick

4 tablespoons olive oil,
   divided, plus additional
   for pan if necessary

2 stalks celery, including
   any leaves, thinly sliced

½ cup thinly sliced shallots
   (3 small shallots)

3 cloves garlic, peeled and
   chopped

8 ounces cremini mushrooms,
   trimmed and thinly sliced
   (about 2½ cups)

1 tablespoon (lightly packed)
   chopped sage

1 tablespoon chopped thyme

¼ cup dry white wine

4 large leaves chard, roughly
   chopped (about 3 cups)

½ cup dried sour cherries or
   dried cranberries, roughly
   chopped

½ cup parsley, roughly
   chopped

½ cup toasted walnuts,
   lightly chopped

1 teaspoon orange zest, orange
   reserved for glaze

(ingredients continue)

I am someone who could have a Thanksgiving dinner 365 days a year. Why do we only get to eat like this on one day? Why can't we have stuffing and turkey and trimmings and gravy and the whole thing on other occasions? Would that make it less special? I suppose it would.

During the holidays there are so many articles and pictures and recipes everyone shares with friends and loved ones—everyone wants to find a nouveau look at this traditional meal. So here is an inspired flavor explosion that with each bite you will be reminded of this very special day, but in a very modern way—it's all in one dish! No sides needed. And as you can guess, I recommend it for any time you get that craving, on any day of the year.

Dry brine the turkey. In a small bowl, combine the sugar, 2½ teaspoons salt, and ½ teaspoon pepper. Sprinkle evenly on both sides of the turkey, cover, and transfer to the refrigerator. Let it brine for at least 4 hours or up to overnight.

Make the stuffing. Heat a large skillet over medium-high heat. Add 2 tablespoons of olive oil, swirl to coat, and add the celery, shallots, and garlic. Season with salt and pepper and cook, stirring, until the vegetables are translucent and softened, adjusting the heat as necessary to prevent browning, about 5 minutes. Add the mushrooms, sage, thyme, and an additional sprinkle of salt. Raise the heat to high and cook, stirring occasionally, until the vegetables begin to turn golden and the mushrooms are tender, about 3 minutes more.

Add the wine, stirring the bottom of the pan to deglaze, and cook until nearly evaporated, about 1 minute. Add the chard and continue to cook, folding to incorporate, until just wilted, 1 to 2 minutes more.

Transfer to a bowl and add the dried fruit, parsley, walnuts, and orange zest. Toss to combine and season to taste with salt and pepper. Let cool completely. (The stuffing can be made up to 1 day in advance. Store in an airtight container in the refrigerator until ready to use.)

Walnut Gremolata (recipe follows)

For the Glaze

½ cup freshly squeezed orange juice, from 1 navel orange

1 tablespoon balsamic vinegar

2 teaspoons tamari (or soy sauce, if not keeping gluten-free)

1 tablespoon water

Make the glaze. In a small pot, combine the orange juice, balsamic vinegar, tamari, and water. Bring to a boil and reduce the heat to maintain a brisk simmer. Cook until the liquid is reduced to a syrupy consistency that can coat the back of a spoon, 8 to 12 minutes. Remove from the heat. (The glaze can be made up to 3 days in advance. Gently rewarm when ready to use.)

Make the roulade. Preheat the oven to 325 degrees. Remove the turkey from the refrigerator and pat dry. On a clean cutting board, lay the turkey flat, cut-side up. Spread 2 cups of the stuffing onto the meat in a thin, even layer, all the way to the edges. Starting from the shortest side, roll the turkey into a tight log.

Cut 5 (14-inch) pieces of butcher string. Lay the roast flat, with the seam side down. Slide the pieces of string underneath the roast, spacing them 1½ inches apart. Tie each string in a knot to secure, starting with the piece in the middle and working your way out to the edges. The knots should hold the roulade in a compact shape, and not be too slack or too tight. Trim the excess string and tuck any bits of stuffing that may have fallen out back into the center. Reserve the remaining stuffing, covered, at room temperature.

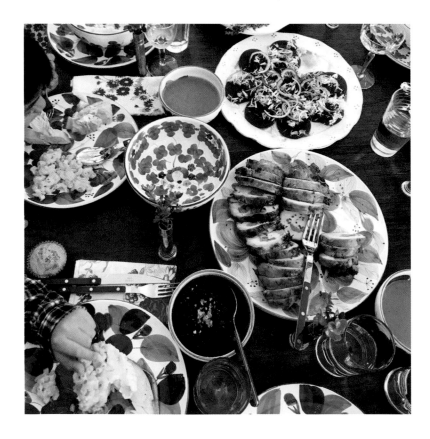

Heat a large, oven-proof skillet over medium-high heat. Add the remaining 2 tablespoons of olive oil, swirl to coat, and add the roulade. Sear, reducing the heat as necessary to avoid burning, until the roast is deeply golden all over, about 2 minutes per side (8 minutes total).

Brush the glaze on all sides of the roulade, and return to the skillet, seam-side down. Add ¼ cup water and transfer to the oven and roast, brushing with glaze every 15 minutes, adding a few tablespoons of water to the pan as necessary to prevent scorching. After 30 minutes, add the reserved stuffing to the pan and spread in an even layer, surrounding the roulade. Continue roasting until an instant-read thermometer inserted into the center reads 150 to 155 degrees, 5 to 15 minutes more, or 40 to 50 minutes total.

Remove the roast from the oven and transfer to a cutting board to rest, 10 to 15 minutes. Lightly cover to keep warm.

Serve. Slice the roulade into ¾-inch slices and divide among serving plates. Top each portion with a spoonful of Walnut Gremolata, and serve immediately.

Walnut Gremolata

YIELD APPROXIMATELY ²/₃ CUP

1 tablespoon olive oil

⅓ cup coarse bread crumbs (to keep things gluten-free, we use bread crumbs made from Base Culture bread)

Kosher salt and freshly ground black pepper

⅓ cup finely chopped toasted walnuts

½ teaspoon lemon zest

¾ teaspoon orange zest

¼ cup parsley, chopped

1 teaspoon thyme, chopped

1 clove garlic, grated

Heat a small skillet over medium heat. Add the olive oil, swirl to coat, and add the bread crumbs. Season with salt and pepper and toast until fragrant, 2 to 3 minutes. Transfer to a bowl and let cool. Add the walnuts, lemon zest, orange zest, parsley, thyme, and garlic. Toss to combine and season to taste with salt and pepper.

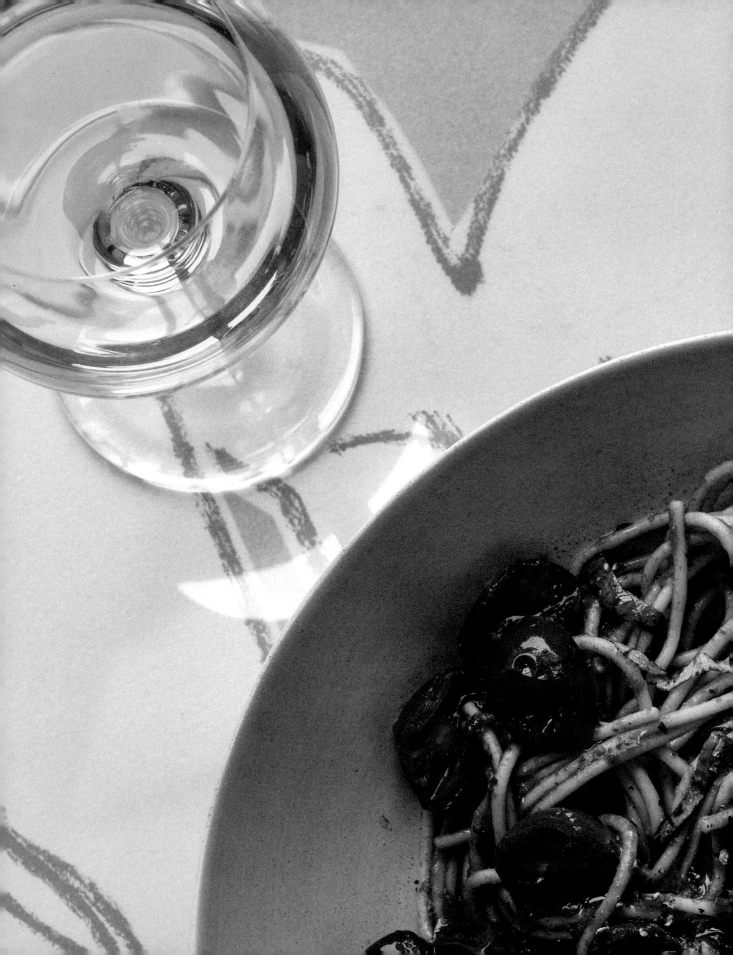

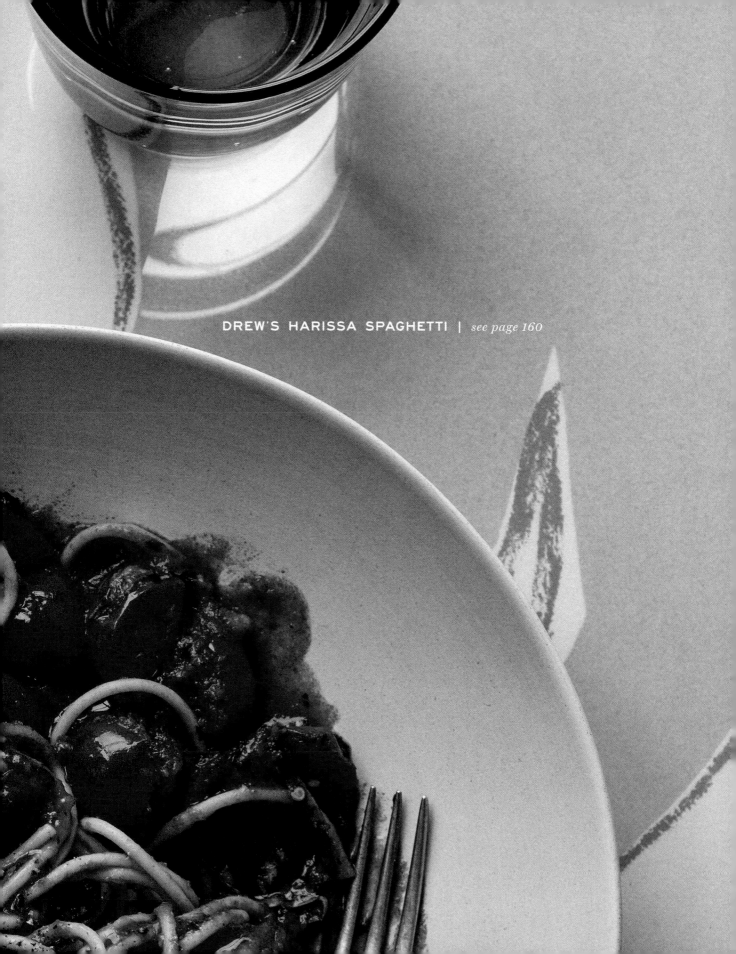

DREW'S HARISSA SPAGHETTI | *see page 160*

Drew's Harissa Spaghetti

SERVES 2

1 (8-ounce) package
chickpea spaghetti
(we recommend Banza)

3 tablespoons olive oil, divided

5 cloves garlic, peeled and
grated

1/4 teaspoon red pepper flakes

1 tablespoon onion powder
(optional)

2 pints cherry tomatoes,
halved

1 tablespoon dried oregano
(optional)

1 tablespoon dried parsley
(optional)

Kosher salt and freshly
ground black pepper

3 tablespoons double-
concentrated tomato paste

2 to 3 tablespoons harissa
paste, plus additional to
taste

1/2 cup chopped basil, plus
additional for serving

I guess if someone was to ask me if I had a signature dish, I'd say this one! Although I'll note that this is a question I never thought I would receive, because until the last few years, my answer would've been "call for takeout." But this is a dish I can confidently whip up anytime, anywhere. I love that it all comes from pantry staples, like canned tomatoes and dried oregano. Or you could make yourself look like a fancy pants and buy fresh cherry tomatoes and fresh basil and simmer that garlic like a real chef! But the key, no matter, is the harissa. It's a Tunisian spice that you squeeze out of a tube, and the result is this smoky and delicious flavor I fell in love with.

Cook the pasta. Bring a large pot of water to a boil over high heat. Season with 2 tablespoons salt. Add the spaghetti and stir to ensure that the pasta does not clump together. Boil until just al dente, 6 to 7 minutes. Reserve 1 cup of the pasta cooking water and drain the noodles. Rinse the chickpea noodles under cold water until completely cool. Set aside.

Make the sauce. Meanwhile, heat a large saucepan over medium-high heat. Add 2 tablespoons of olive oil and swirl to coat. Add the garlic, red pepper flakes, and onion powder, if using. Sauté, stirring, until the garlic is fragrant, 30 seconds to 1 minute. Do not let brown. Add the cherry tomatoes and dried herbs, if using, and season with salt and pepper. Continue cooking until the tomatoes begin to break down, 4 to 5 minutes. Add the tomato paste and harissa paste and cook for 3 minutes more. Taste the sauce and season with salt, pepper, and additional harissa paste, if desired. (The pasta sauce can be made up to 3 days in advance. Store, covered, in the refrigerator before reheating in a skillet.)

Serve. Add the pasta to the sauce, along with 1 to 2 tablespoons of pasta water to thin, if necessary. The sauce should be thick and concentrated, but just loose enough to coat the noodles easily. Cook for 1 minute more, tossing to combine. Add the chopped basil, gently fold to combine, and divide among serving plates. Serve immediately, topping each portion with a drizzle of olive oil and additional basil.

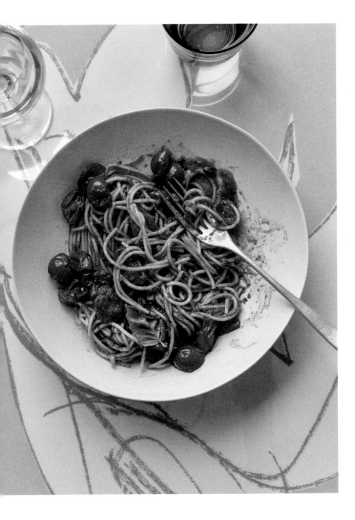
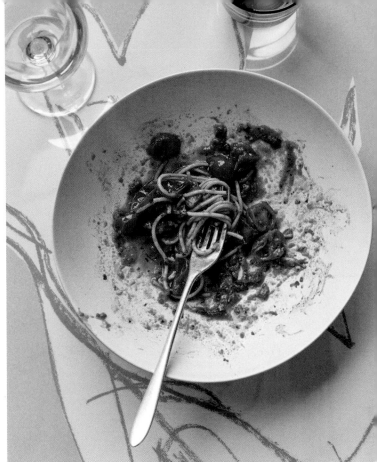
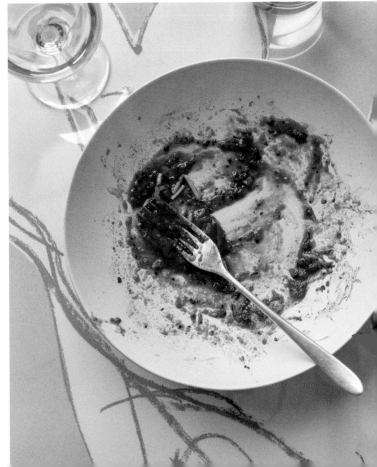

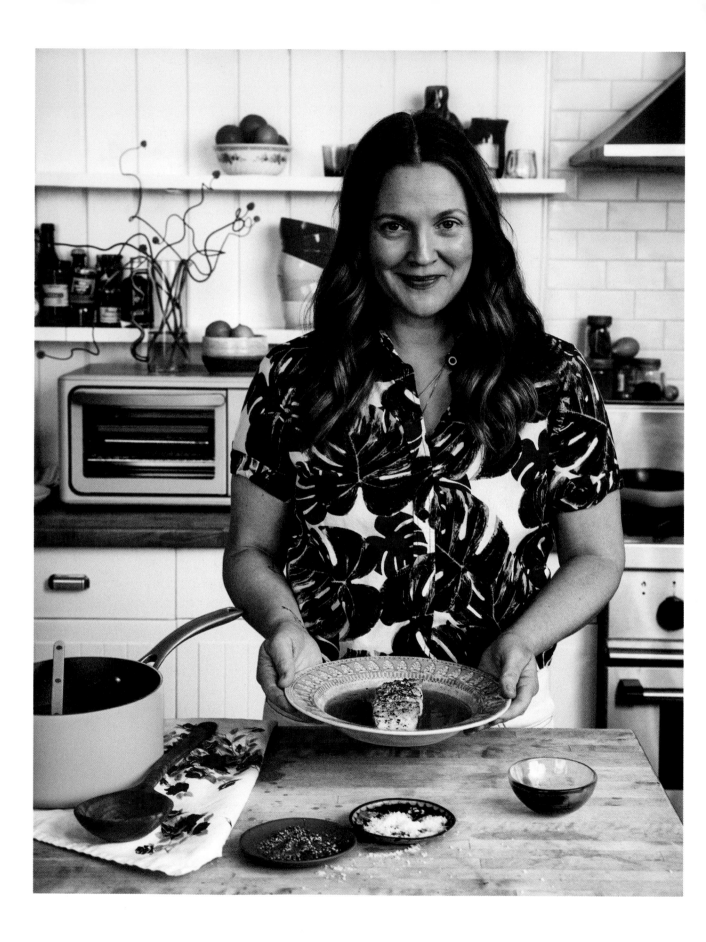

Seared Halibut with Saffron Broth

SERVES 2

1 shallot, peeled and sliced

1 small or ½ medium leek, rinsed well, cut into 2-inch pieces

1 clove garlic, peeled and sliced

Kosher salt and freshly ground black pepper

1 roma tomato, roughly chopped

1 stalk celery, including leaves, cut into 2-inch pieces

4 ounces fresh shiitake mushrooms (about 2 cups) or 10 dried shiitakes (about ¾ ounce)

½ bunch parsley

8 sprigs thyme

2 bay leaves

1 teaspoon whole black peppercorns

4 cups water

1 generous pinch saffron

Freshly ground black pepper

2 halibut fillets, skin off (5 to 6 ounces each)

2 teaspoons olive oil

Flaky sea salt (we love Maldon), for serving

I love this fish dish! Cooking fish used to intimidate me, but with these tips, I have been able to tackle this recipe easily.

First, make sure you buy the freshest fish you can. If you can chat with the person at the grocery store, or the fish-monger, to see what is best and freshest, even better. Since there are so few components in this recipe, you really want that fish to be a star. We like to use halibut for this, but you can substitute with other lean white fish, like cod. Just like our tip for cooking steak (page 175), a thicker fillet will give you a little more wiggle room for error when cooking your fish, so if you don't feel as confident yet about cooking the fish, I definitely recommend going with a slightly thicker fillet. Second, when cooking the fish, make sure you pat the fillet dry—moisture will cause the fillet to stick to the pan and you definitely don't want that! I love to use my fish spatula in this recipe to flip and serve. If you don't have one, I definitely recommend it; it's one of my favorite kitchen tools. And it's not only for fish! We use it for pancakes, cookies, and even when flipping grilled cheese sandwiches!

The dish is finished out with one of my favorite broths, and it gets a little extra special love in the recipe with the addition of saffron. (If cooking for one, reduce the fillet to one piece of fish. We recommend making the full recipe of the broth, which can be sipped on its own, or can be frozen up to 1 month.)

Make the broth. In a medium pot, combine the shallot, leek, garlic, tomato, celery, mushrooms, parsley, thyme, bay leaves, peppercorns, ½ teaspoon salt, and water. Bring to a boil, then adjust heat to maintain a brisk boil until the liquid is reduced by one-fourth, 20 to 25 minutes. Strain the broth through a fine-mesh strainer into another pot. Discard the solids. Add the saffron threads to the broth, season to taste with salt and pepper, and keep warm. (The broth can be made ahead of time and kept in the refrigerator in an airtight container, covered, for up to 3 days or frozen for up to 1 month.)

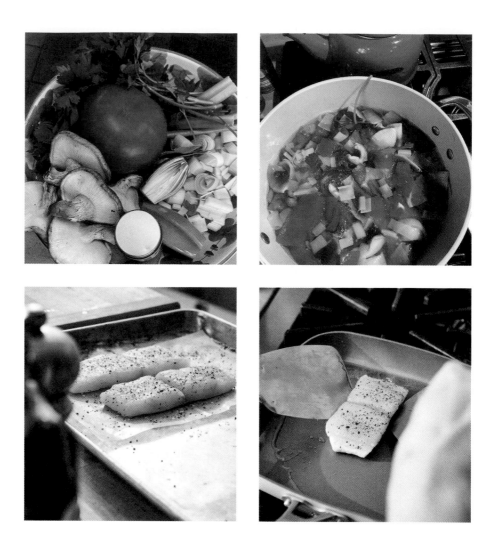

Sear the fish. Pat the fish dry with a paper towel. (You want to make sure there is as little moisture as possible on the fish's surface to avoid sticking to the pan.) Season both sides of the fish with salt and pepper. Heat a medium nonstick skillet over medium heat, add the 2 teaspoons of olive oil, and swirl to coat. As soon as the oil is shimmering, add the fish. Let sear, undisturbed, until lightly golden on the underside, about 5 minutes. Flip the fillets and continue to cook until just cooked through, about 2 minutes more. Remove the skillet from the heat and let the fish sit in the skillet for carryover cooking, 1 minute more.

Serve. Place each of the fillets in individual bowls, golden cooked-side up. Ladle 1 cup of broth around the fish so that the fish is only partially submerged. Garnish with freshly ground black pepper, flaky sea salt, and serve.

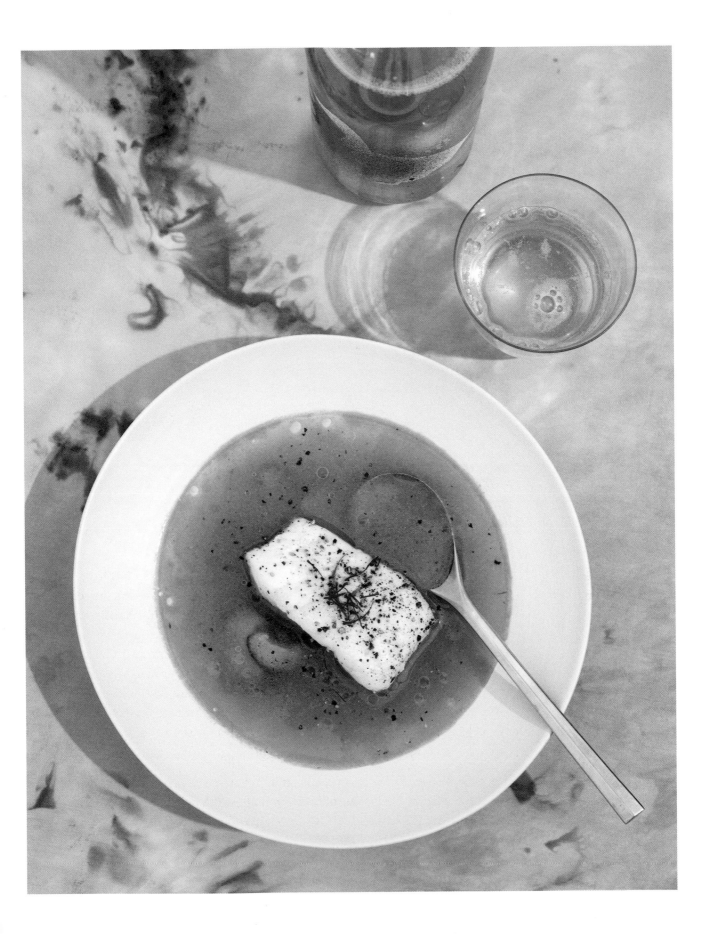

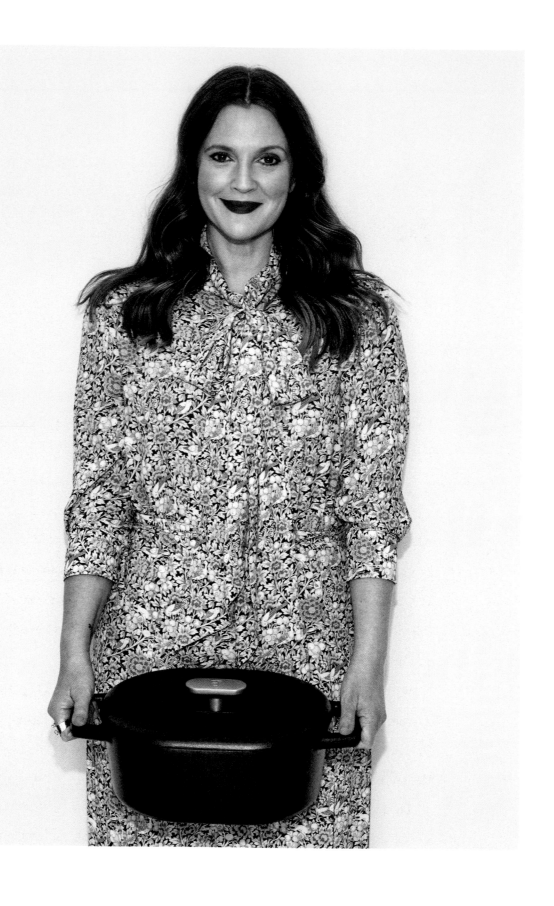

Beautiful Cookware

Beautiful: the story of reimagining how to live in your kitchen . . . because that's really what it was for me.

A man named Shae Hong asked me if I wanted to start a company. We became good friends and realized that our core values as humans aligned, and that deciding what we wanted to make for people was coming into focus as well. I basically took on this project as the lead in the design department. And I was able to collaborate with a team of geniuses who had tremendous experience, having worked at all the major design and manufacturing companies, and could guide us through the technicalities of what was possible.

We challenged ourselves for months. Missed deadlines because I kept saying, "No one needs more stuff! This has to be different or it doesn't matter anyway!" I wanted to create an aesthetic that was new to me. I challenged myself to get out of my own design comfort zone and look to the future—*timeless* is not an overrated word.

I tried to give my cookware line the same spirit as my TV show, trying to re-create nostalgia and comfort, reminding us of the way we grew up, while still embracing

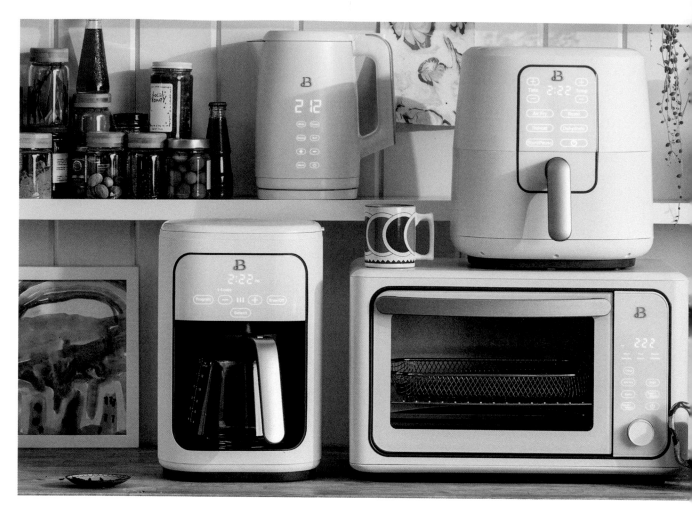

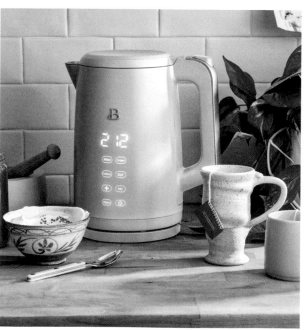

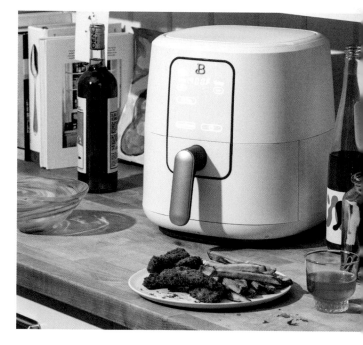

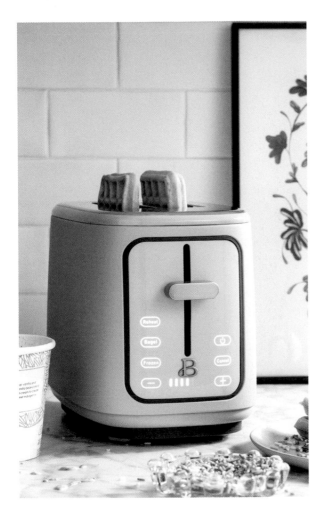

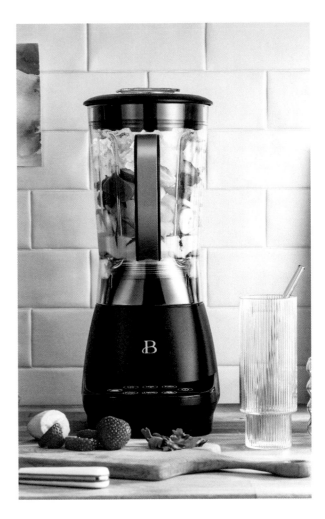

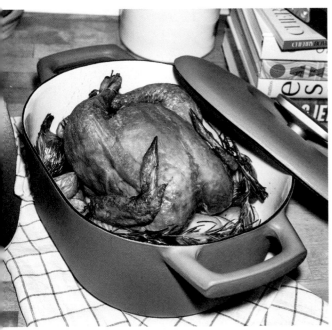

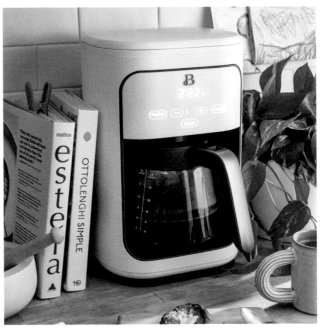

the future. We must innovate. And 2020 certainly asked us all to look at everything differently. That year affected every element of my life—as it did for everyone else's. I think of the past as a bit old and dusty, and I fear the future feeling cold and too modern. I am trying to find the pretty little middle in all the many endeavors I am lucky enough to be a part of. So in the case of focusing on the kitchen, I thought about function as well as sleekness.

I asked myself why all appliances have to be black or silver. To me, that doesn't feel feminine. But then I didn't want it to be overly girlie, either. I told myself, "Think *timeless*. Innovate. And make it something that can look gender neutral and . . . beautiful." And that became the name! Because life and our surroundings are wonderful focal points for beauty. When it comes to the kitchen, most of the things are also out in plain sight! We are forced to look at our countertop appliances every day.

We actually use gadgets; we grab them by the hand. It's all so interactive, both visually and practically. But then the team helped me find a way to remove knobs, dials, and all the stuff that makes kitchen appliances a bit frenzied. I asked if we could bury all the mess in a new way, make it all touch screen, so that only when we are using an item do we then see how it functions. Let's go forward into the future and find what is possible in the way of technology.

Which also leads me to function. These products don't just look a certain way . . . they work incredibly well, too! The truth is, they are made by some of the best in the business and I am confident in the happiness in the result. I believe people will use all of our products and truly be blown away. Oh yeah, one more thing: we also agreed as a team that the prices should never break the bank. That is my mission with all things I am associated with. I am here to provide amazing products at a different price point. That crusade alone is worth everything to me.

This company is our labor of love, to make your kitchen a true place of beauty. That's what the "Beautiful" is all about. YOU! Because *you* deserve to feel that feeling. Make every day pretty!!!!!

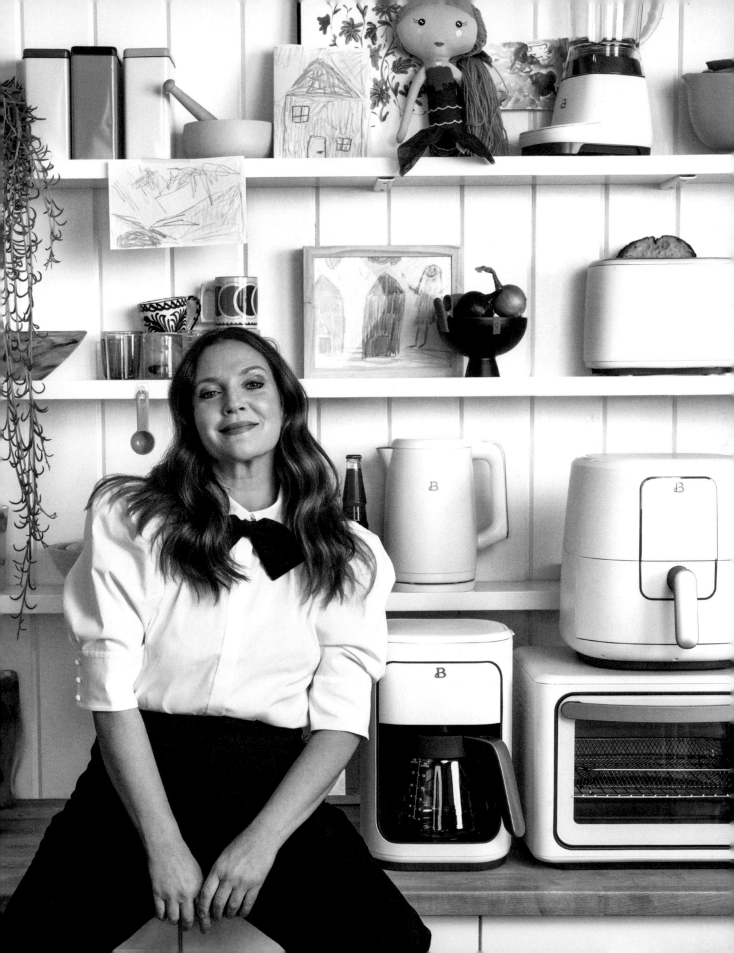

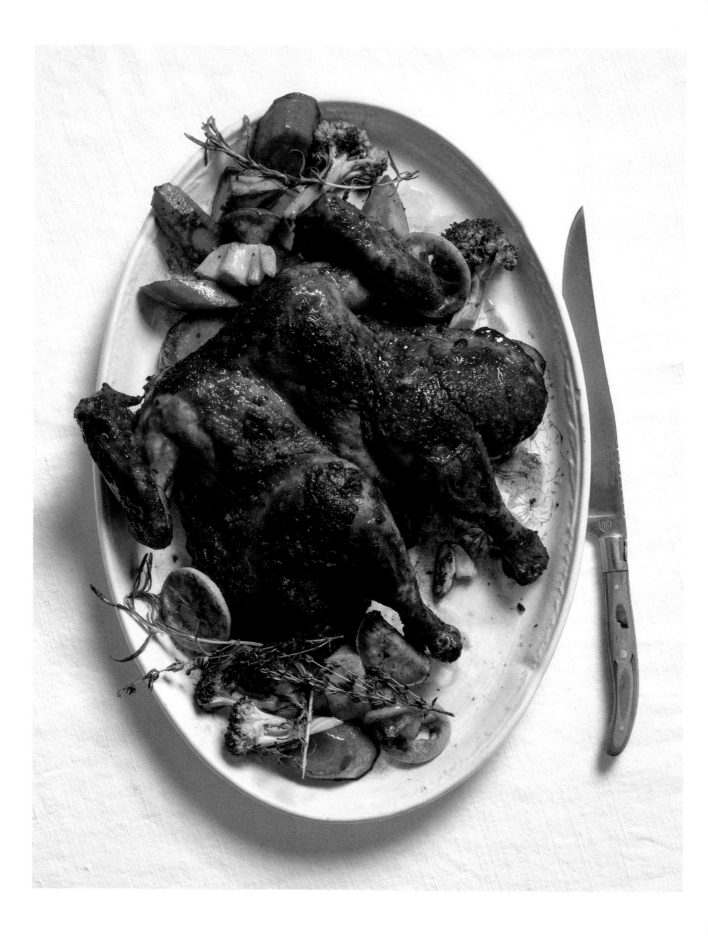

Frankie and Olive's Roast Chicken

SERVES 3 TO 4

½ tablespoon sweet paprika

1 teaspoon onion powder

1 teaspoon garlic powder

Kosher salt and freshly
ground black pepper

1 whole chicken (3½ to 4
pounds), spatchcocked

3 cloves garlic, divided

1 lemon, zested and cut
into ¼-inch slices, plus
additional lemon wedges
for serving

3 tablespoons unsalted butter,
softened

1 carrot, scrubbed and cut into
2-inch pieces

1 head broccoli, florets cut
into 2-inch pieces, stems
peeled and cut into 2-inch
pieces

1 medium sweet potato,
scrubbed and cut into
1½-inch chunks

8 sprigs thyme

1 (4-inch) sprig rosemary,
broken into 2 or 3 pieces

2 tablespoons olive oil

This roast chicken is a weekly tradition at my house, and it's one of the first things Pilar made for the girls. Olive goes in for the drumstick, and Frankie the breast; always a little something for everyone.

A few tips: spatchcocking the chicken helps the chicken cook more evenly and reduces the cooking time, too. If you've never spatchcocked a chicken before—have no fear! It is way easier to do than to say. All you need are some sharp kitchen scissors, and you're all set. Also, we recommend seasoning your bird in advance—up to 1 day. This produces an extra tasty (and crispy-skinned) roast chicken.

Got leftovers? No problem! The fully cooked chicken will keep in the refrigerator for up to three days and can be used to make chicken noodle soup, chicken salad, or chicken tacos. Yum!

Make the rub. In a small bowl, combine the paprika, onion powder, garlic powder, 1 tablespoon plus 1 teaspoon salt, and ½ teaspoon pepper.

Season the bird. Place the chicken on a cutting board. Sprinkle half of the spice mix in between the skin and the meat of the thighs, drumsticks, and breasts. With the remaining spice mix, season the chicken all over, this time focusing on the skin and the underside. It may seem like you have a lot of spice mix, but if you thoroughly coat the meat and skin all over, you should use it all up.

Place the chicken on a large plate and transfer to the refrigerator, uncovered, skin-side up, until ready to roast, at least 1 hour and up to 1 day in advance. This produces a well-seasoned chicken and helps the skin crisp.

Make the compound butter. In a small bowl, grate 1 clove of the garlic, then add the lemon zest and butter. Mix until smooth.

Roast the chicken. Preheat the oven to 475 degrees. Remove the chicken from the refrigerator and let it sit at room temperature for 30 minutes. Pat it dry. Place the chicken in the center of a rimmed sheet pan, breast-side up, and tuck the wing tips behind the tops of the breasts to prevent burning.

Using a spoon, or your hands, gently stuff half of the compound butter underneath the skin of the breast meat. Rub the remaining compound butter all over the chicken.

Smash the remaining 2 cloves garlic. In a large bowl, combine the lemon slices, smashed garlic, carrot, broccoli, sweet potato, thyme, and rosemary. Drizzle with olive oil and toss to coat thoroughly. Season with salt and pepper. Scatter the vegetables around the chicken, tucking a few onion or sweet potato pieces underneath the chicken, so as not to overcrowd the perimeter of the pan.

Transfer the sheet pan to the oven, legs first, which will encourage the dark and light meat to cook at an even rate. Immediately reduce the oven temperature to 425.

Roast for 35 to 40 minutes, rotating the pan halfway through, until the chicken skin is deeply golden and an instant-read thermometer reads 160 to 165 degrees when inserted into the thickest part of the thigh or breast.

Serve. Let it rest for 10 minutes before carving. Serve with roasted vegetables, pan juices, and extra lemon wedges on the side.

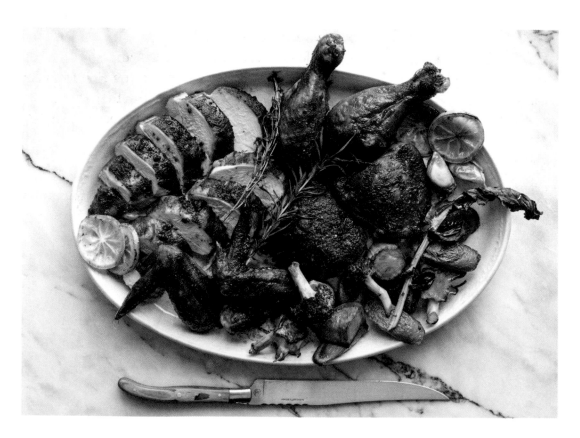

Peppery Steak with Cranberry Agrodolce

SERVES 2

For the Steak

1 (1-pound) New York strip steak, about 1½ inches thick

Kosher salt

2 tablespoons black peppercorns

1 tablespoon avocado oil, plus additional for searing

Flaky sea salt (we love Maldon), for serving

Lightly chopped fresh tarragon, for serving (optional)

For the Cranberry Agrodolce

2 heaping tablespoons finely chopped shallots, from 1 small shallot

⅓ cup balsamic vinegar

3 tablespoons dried cranberries, roughly chopped

1 teaspoon honey

¼ cup water

1 heaping teaspoon dijon mustard

I love a good steak once in a while, and I really wanted to include one in this book to share how easy it is to cook—if I can make it, so can you!

A few tips from Pilar about your steak: you want to buy a steak with good marbling all throughout. Fat is flavor, and a well-marbled piece of meat will have better flavor and moisture. *Yum.* She recommends buying a steak that is at least 1½ inches thick; a thicker steak will develop that beautiful, toasty, crunchy crust on the steak, without overcooking. A thicker piece of meat also gives you a little more wiggle room for error. Season your meat in advance, if possible, at least 45 minutes and up to 2 days (just keep it on a rack over a plate in the fridge if seasoning longer than 45 minutes). We use a New York strip for this because it cooks up so quickly and has the tenderness of the fillet but the flavor of a rib eye. Last tip: always use your instant-read thermometer. Take the guesswork out of how cooked your meat is!

Agrodolce is an Italian sweet-and-sour condiment. It pairs perfectly here as a side to the rich steak, but we imagine it could go really well with other things, too, like roasted brussels sprouts or a hearty piece of fish.

Preheat your oven to 400 degrees.

Season the steak. At least 45 minutes before cooking, place your steak on a plate and season all sides liberally with 2 teaspoons of salt. Set aside, uncovered.

Meanwhile, in a mortar and pestle, crush the black peppercorns, allowing for variations in texture and size, coarse and fine. Transfer the peppercorns to a dinner plate. Pat the steak dry. Rub a small amount of avocado oil on the surface of the steak and lay it on top of the crushed peppercorns, pressing lightly so they adhere. Repeat with the other side.

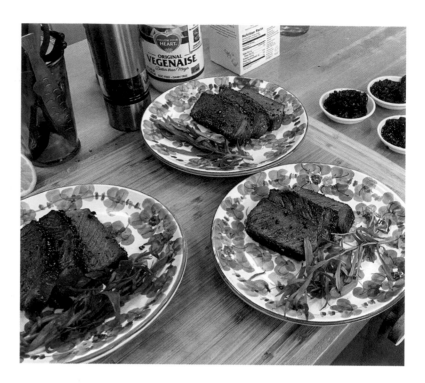

Cook the steak. Turn on the exhaust fan (it will get smoky!). Preheat an oven-safe skillet over medium-high heat. (Note: If using a cast-iron skillet, we recommend cooking over medium heat as the peppercorns may toast more quickly.) When the pan is hot (you can check it by sprinkling a drop of water on it—it should sizzle immediately), add 1 tablespoon avocado oil and swirl to coat. Carefully add the steak and let sear, undisturbed, for 3 minutes. Flip and continue searing for an additional 3 minutes, adding additional avocado oil if the skillet seems dry. Be careful at all times to preserve as many of the peppercorns as possible on the surface of the steak. Carefully prop the steak on its side, fat-side down, and continue to sear, rendering the fat, about 1 minute more.

Take the temperature. Insert an instant-read thermometer into the thickest part of the steak. If you like a rare steak, it may read 120 degrees at this point, and if so, you can set it aside to rest on the cutting board. (Please keep in mind that steak cuts and pans can vary. For a perfectly cooked steak, according to your desired doneness, always use an instant-read thermometer.)

Finish in the oven. Transfer the pan to the oven and continue cooking, until you reach your desired doneness: 125 to 130 degrees for medium rare (4 to 6 minutes in the oven), 140 to 145 degrees for medium (6 to 8 minutes in the oven).

Remove the pan from the oven, transfer the steak to a cutting board, and let it rest for 10 minutes before cutting.

While the steak is resting, make the sauce. Place the shallots, balsamic vinegar, cranberries, honey, water, and a pinch of salt in a small pot. Place over medium heat, bring to a boil, and reduce heat to maintain a brisk simmer. Let cook, swirling the pot occasionally, until slightly thickened, about 4 minutes. Remove from the heat and immediately stir in the mustard. Check for seasoning.

Serve. Slice the steak to desired thickness. Season with flaky sea salt and garnish with fresh tarragon leaves, if using. Serve with Cranberry Agrodolce on the side.

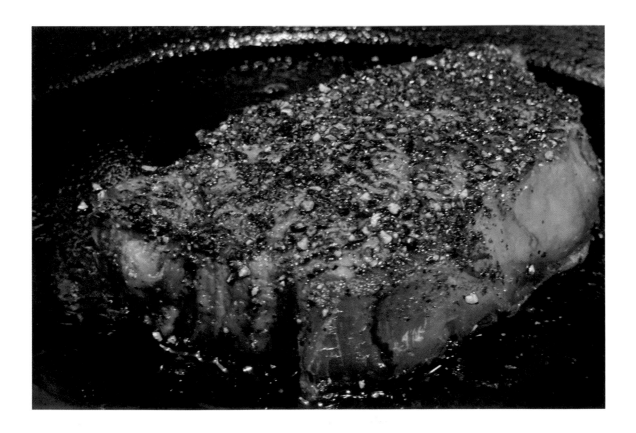

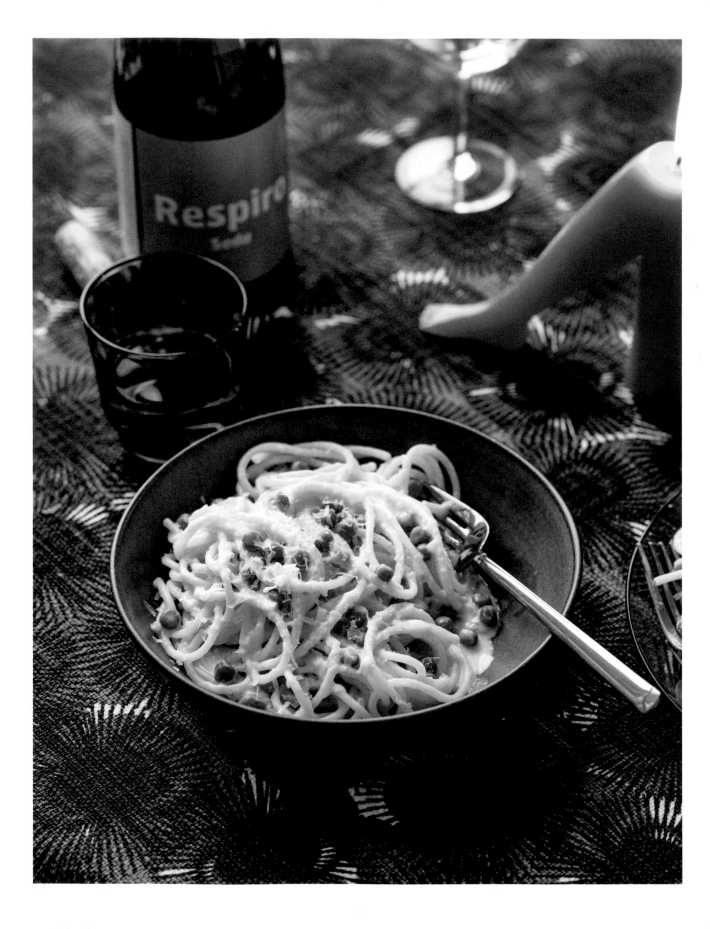

8 ounces bucatini (or linguine or spaghetti)

Kosher salt

1 tablespoon unsalted butter

2 cloves garlic, peeled and roughly chopped

1 lemon, zested and juiced, plus additional lemon juice for serving

1 cup fresh or frozen peas

1 tablespoon finely grated Parmigiano Reggiano, plus additional for serving

¼ cup mascarpone

Pasta al Limone with Peas (Two Ways)

Classic Version

When Pilar and I started dreaming up this book, one of my original ideas was to do recipes of my favorite dishes side by side with a vegan and gluten-free spin on it. And these two recipes are our takes on that.

Pasta al Limone, how do I love thee? Let me count the ways. It has bucatini pasta (one of my favorites! But feel free to substitute your favorite long pasta), not one but two types of cheese, and peas. I live for peas, the more the better. The vegan version uses our Lemony Cashew Cream (page 182), finished with peas. Always peas. I love both versions and they are each delicious in their own right.

Keep in mind, this pasta dish waits for no one! Make sure you (or your guests) are seated and ready to eat before serving the dish. It is best hot and inhaled within minutes.

Cook the noodles. Bring a large pot of salted water to a boil over high heat. Add the bucatini and continue to cook, stirring occasionally, until just under al dente, about 1 minute less than the recommended cooking time on the package. Reserve 1 cup of pasta water and set aside. Drain the noodles and return to the pot.

Make the sauce. While the pasta cooks, heat a medium skillet over medium heat. Add the butter and let it melt. As soon as the foaming subsides, add the garlic to the pan. Season with salt and sauté, stirring, until aromatic and softened, about 1 minute. Do not brown. Add the lemon juice, half of the zest, ¼ cup of the reserved pasta cooking water, and the peas. Bring to a boil and reduce, stirring constantly, about 30 seconds. Working as quickly as you can, add the drained noodles to the sauce. Fold in Parmigiano Reggiano and the mascarpone and toss, adding additional pasta water by the tablespoon, until the sauce is velvety and the pasta is very generously coated. The noodles should feel *nearly* overdressed, as pasta will continue absorbing the sauce as it sits.

Serve. Top with the remaining lemon zest, additional Parmigiano Reggiano, and a squeeze of fresh lemon.

Gluten-Free/Vegan Version

SERVES 2

8 ounces gluten-free spaghetti (we recommend Banza)

Kosher salt

1 tablespoon unsalted vegan butter (we love Miyoko's)

2 cloves garlic, peeled and roughly chopped

1 lemon, zested and juiced, plus additional for serving

1 cup fresh or frozen peas

¼ cup Lemony Cashew Cream (recipe follows)

1½ teaspoons nutritional yeast, plus additional for serving

Flaky sea salt (we love Maldon), for serving

Cook the noodles. Bring a large pot of salted water to a boil over high heat. Add the gluten-free spaghetti and continue to cook, stirring occasionally, until just under al dente, about 9 minutes. Reserve 1 cup of pasta water and set aside. Drain the noodles and rinse under cold water until completely cool. Set aside.

Make the sauce. While the pasta cooks, heat a medium skillet over medium heat. Add the vegan butter and melt. As soon as the bubbles subside, swirl to coat, and add the garlic. Season with salt and sauté, stirring, until aromatic and softened, about 1 minute. Do not let it brown. Add the lemon juice, half of the zest, ¼ cup of the reserved pasta cooking water, and the peas. Bring to a boil and let reduce, stirring occasionally, about 30 seconds. Turn off the heat. Working quickly, add the Lemony Cashew Cream (page 182) and the nutritional yeast, stir until fully combined, and add the pasta. Add additional pasta water by the tablespoon, folding gently to incorporate until the sauce is velvety and the pasta is very generously coated. The noodles should feel *nearly* overdressed, as the pasta will continue absorbing the sauce as it sits.

Serve. Top with the remaining lemon zest, a sprinkle of nutritional yeast, flaky sea salt, and a fresh squeeze of lemon.

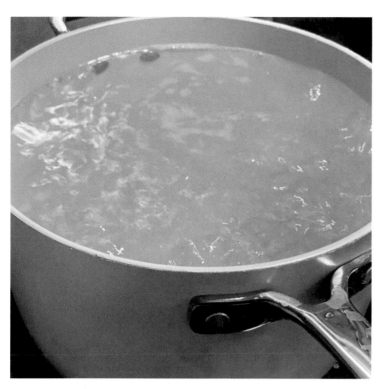

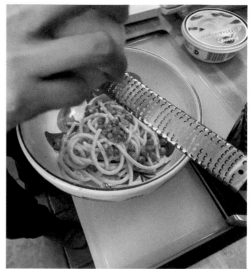

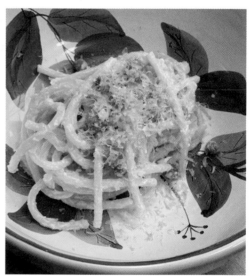

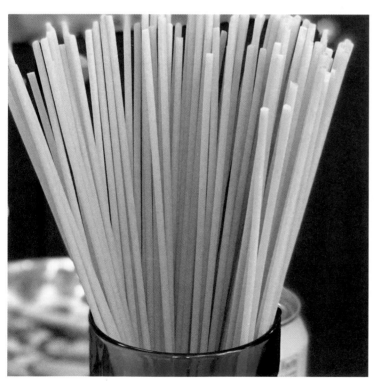

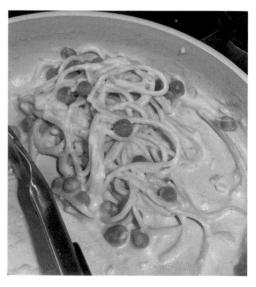

Lemony Cashew Cream

3 ounces (heaping ½ cup) raw cashews, soaked in water for 1 hour and drained

⅓ cup water

1 tablespoon freshly squeezed lemon juice

2 teaspoons dijon mustard

Kosher salt

Make the cream. Combine the cashews, water, lemon juice, mustard, and ½ teaspoon salt in a blender. (An immersion blender also works!) Blend the mixture until very smooth and creamy, scraping down the sides of the bowl as necessary. Cashew cream can keep, covered, in the refrigerator, for up to 5 days.

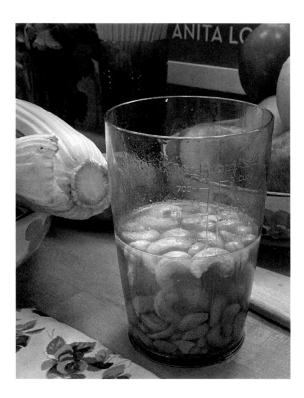
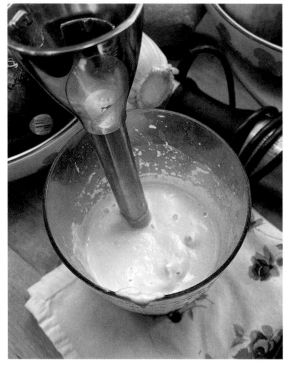

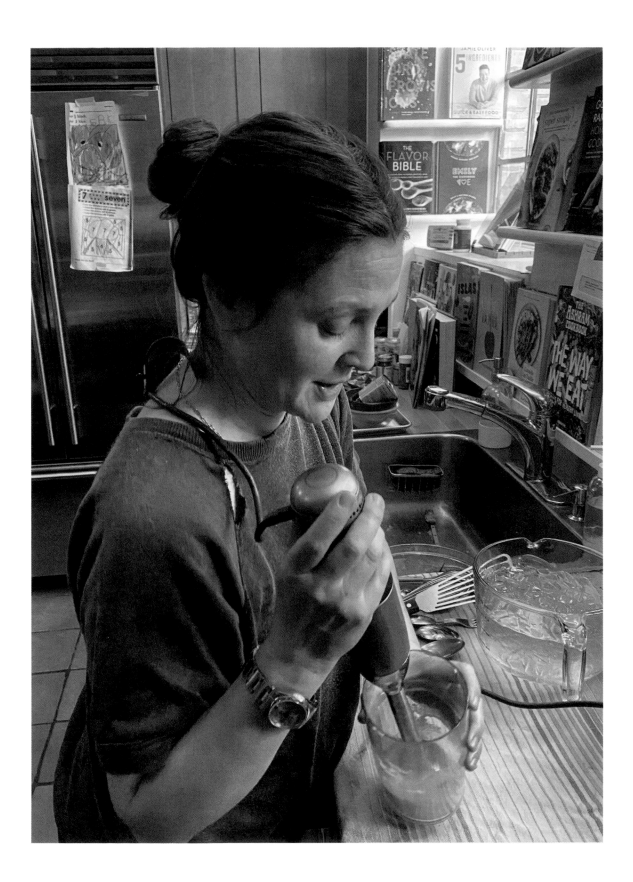

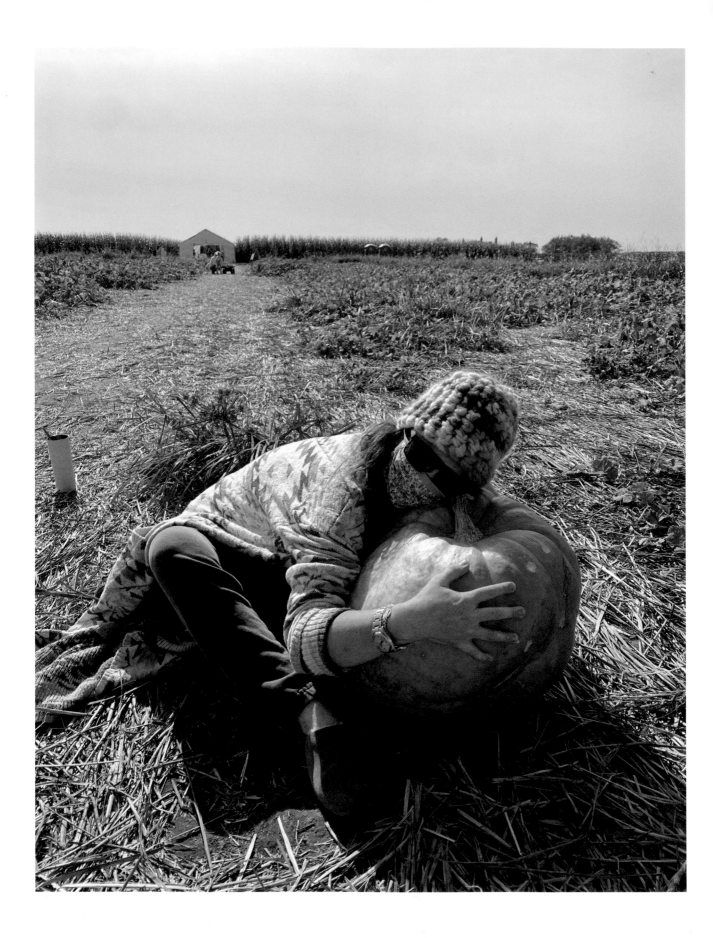

Oh, the Holidays!

Drew: I start with themes. I love a costume party. I love a themed party. I love holidays. We decorate our entryway for Easter, and Valentine's Day, and St. Patrick's Day, and Earth Day. Fourth of July!

Pilar: You guys really do it up well! That little vestibule is a showcase!

Drew: Halloween is the best! We go all out. The most terrifying . . . Our entryway is only about three feet by four feet . . .

Pilar: But you guys really pack it in!

Drew: We do. Every holiday, we try to be really theme oriented. As far as birthdays, I really want to know what the girls' themes are. But when you're entertaining for kids, you have to really think about the adults, too. Get them beverages, find out what they like to eat. Make sure there's a good balance of refreshments for all ages. As a parent who takes kids to birthday parties, I've noticed it's always really kid focused. And the parents are sipping apple juice boxes.

Pilar: You really make it a point to take care of everyone. Not just for holidays but for birthdays. You're always going the extra mile to figure out "What would this person want? How can we make them feel special?"

Drew: I think about activities also. I love a game at a dinner party. I love activities happening for kids' parties, like pictures and crafts. Animals visiting! I love busying people. If you're going to decide to entertain, make sure that people have enough food and drink to feel comfortable enjoying both. That's a very fortunate thing to be able to do, and I never take it for granted. But as a host and entertainer of people through lunches and dinner parties, and birthdays and holidays—I don't want to be excessive, but I want people to feel the abundance of the moment in a celebratory way.

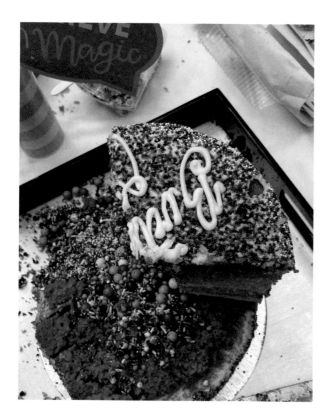
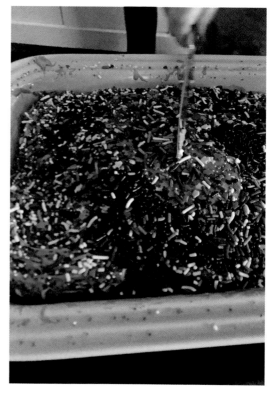

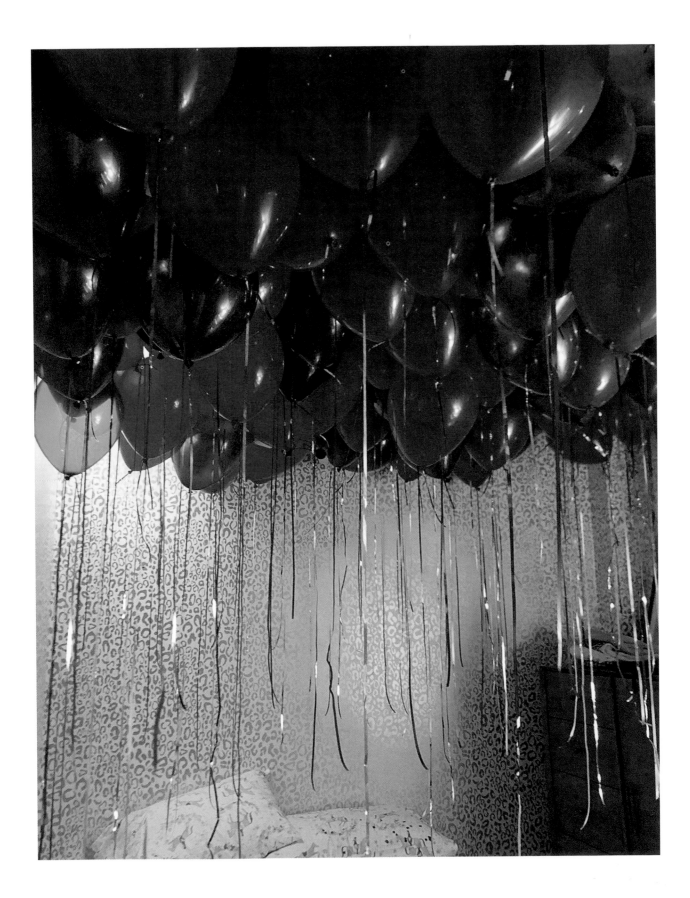

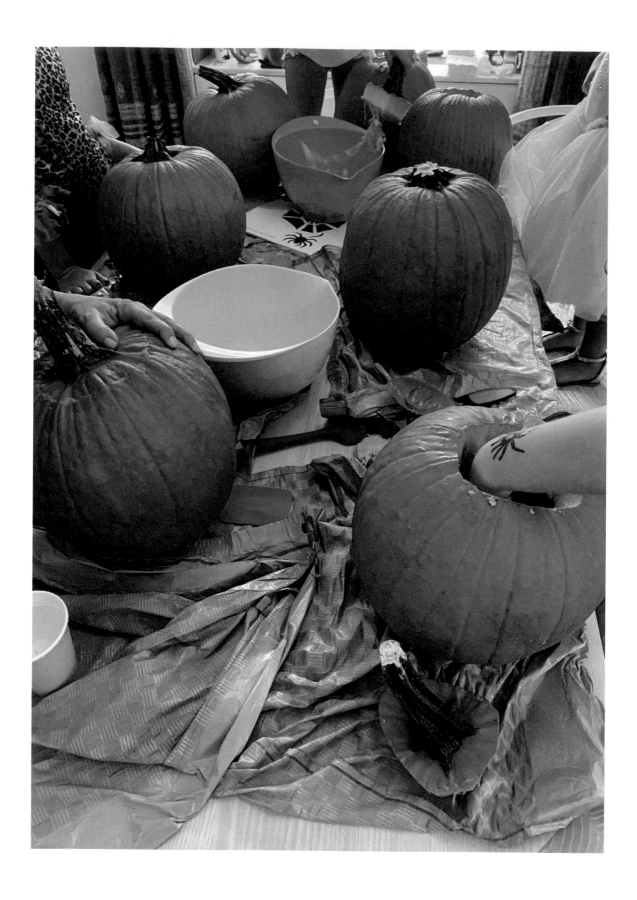

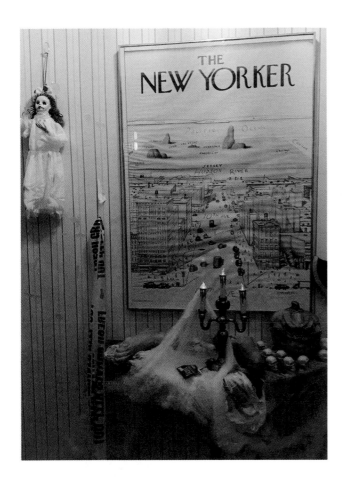

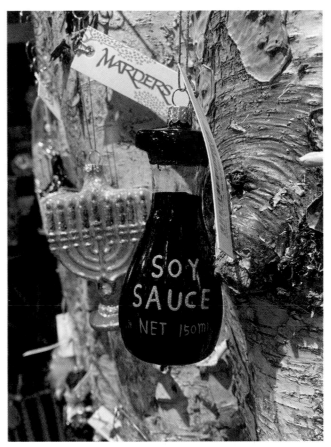

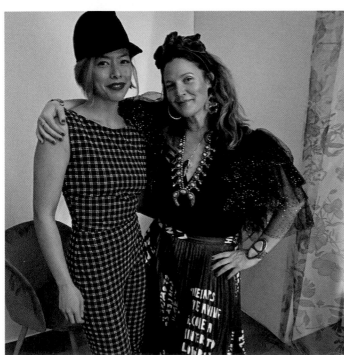

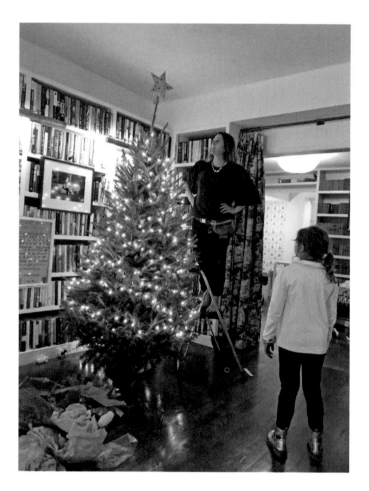

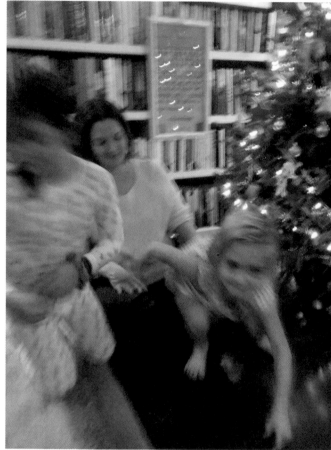

Pilar: What's so wonderful about this house, too, is that food is always on offer. I feel like anyone who walks in, you say, "Have you eaten? Can we offer you something?" It never has to be fancy. But you're just opening your home and offering people something, and that's wonderful.

Drew: And I'm constantly trying to feed two kids and have healthy snacks, and figure out their developing appetites. I think that's another way for me to be a caretaker, to have food and drinks for everybody. I'm a very old Jewish grandmother that way. "Sit down, darling. Have you eaten?"

Pilar: And that's so true to your nature. You're a deeply caring person. You make people feel good that way.

Drew: And not to be maudlin, but I grew up in a home that did not have real meals; that was replaced with travel and eating around the world. I didn't grow up in a home where we sat around a dinner table, so that was something I wanted to pursue as an adult—to have a home that was flowing with food and life. Because that was the antithesis of my childhood. But all that stuff wasn't missing; it was replaced with worldly experience. And I wouldn't trade that for anything.

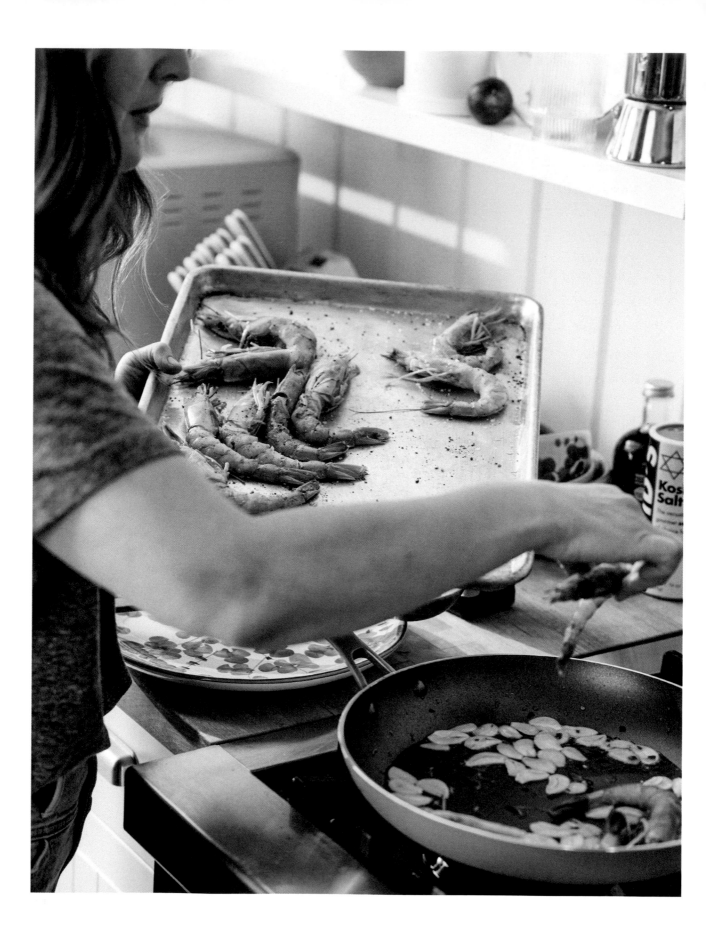

Stovetop Scampi

SERVES 2 TO 4

1 pound (U/10 or U/12) head-
    on shrimp, peeled with
    inner tract removed, heads
    and tails left on

Kosher salt and freshly
    ground black pepper

2 tablespoons olive oil

4 cloves garlic, peeled and
    thinly sliced

½ teaspoon red pepper flakes

3 tablespoons butter, divided

⅓ cup dry white wine

2 lemons, plus additional
    lemon wedges for serving

¼ cup roughly chopped flat-
    leaf parsley

I love shrimp. Full stop. And this is my favorite scampi rec-ipe of all time. It is ridiculously simple and out-of-control delicious. The most complicated part (which I've discov-ered I'm actually really good at—who knew?) is peeling the shrimp!

In the United States shrimp are sold according to piece per pound—so when you're at the store and see U/15, or U/10, that means there are fewer than 15 pieces of shrimp per pound or fewer than 10 pieces of shrimp per pound, respectively. The lower the number, the larger the shrimp. For this recipe, I love using head-on U/10 shrimp. Head-and shells-on typically mean they're fresher, and the heads add soooo much flavor to the sauce.

That being said, I totally get that head-on is not for ev-eryone, and you can substitute peeled and deveined 16/20 shrimp here, and they will cook at pretty much the same rate as the recipe below. This is definitely a special treat. Lemony sunshine, glorious shrimp, and garlic buttah—treat yourself!

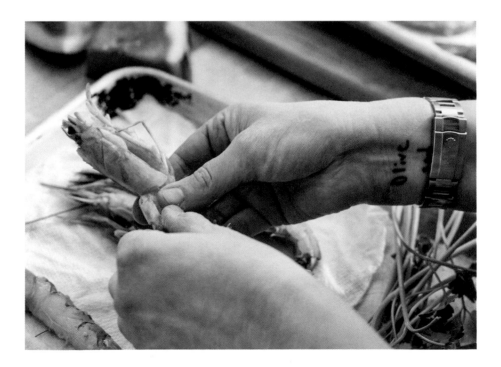

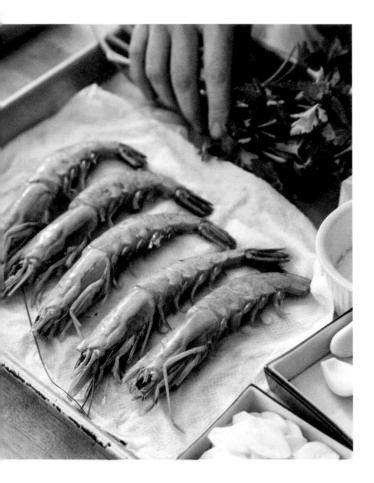

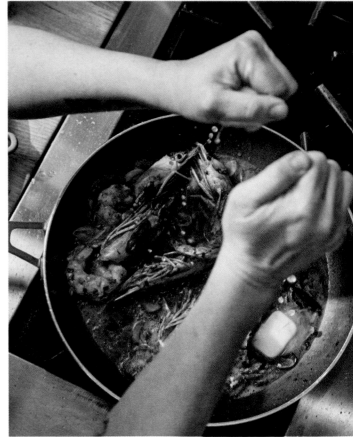

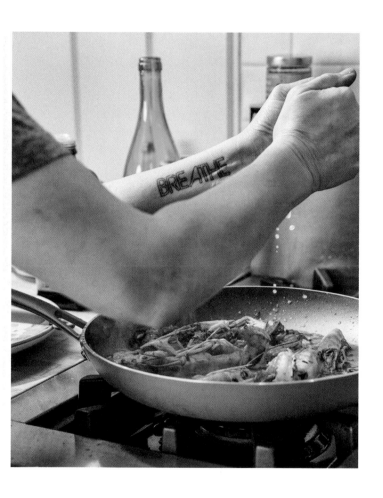

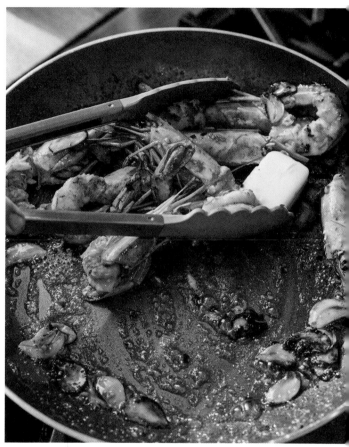

Cook the shrimp. Season one side of the shrimp with salt and pepper.

Heat a large skillet (big enough to fit all your shrimp in one layer) over medium heat. Add the olive oil and swirl to coat. Add the garlic and red pepper flakes and cook until slightly translucent and the oil is infused with the garlic–red pepper flavor, about 1 minute. (If you prefer less toasted garlic, remove the garlic slices now with a slotted spoon and set aside for later.)

Raise the heat to medium-high. Add the shrimp, seasoned-side down, in a single layer. Season the second side of shrimp (the side facing you) with salt and pepper. Cook, gently shaking the pan occasionally, just until the shrimp begin to change color and have some golden spots on the undersides, about 1½ minutes. Carefully flip the shrimp, keeping the heads and bodies intact. Add 2 tablespoons butter, the white wine, and the juice from 1 lemon to the pan. Continue cooking, shaking the pan, until the shrimp is just cooked through, about 1½ minutes more. Remove the shrimp to a plate and cover. (If you removed the garlic earlier, add it back into the pan now.) Let the sauce continue to reduce, about 1 minute more, stirring occasionally. Check for seasoning. Add more lemon or butter, if needed, whisking to emulsify. The sauce should be bright but balanced by a rich, buttery backbone. If too acidic, continue reducing in 30-second increments.

Serve. Turn off the heat. Pour the finished sauce on top of the shrimp and top with the parsley. Serve with lemon wedges on the side.

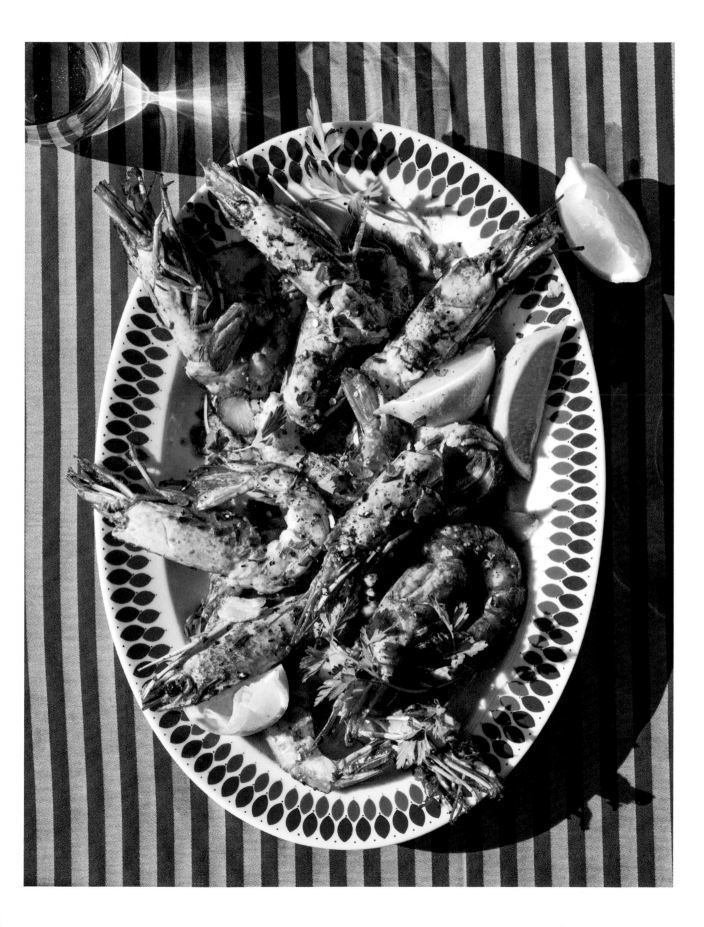

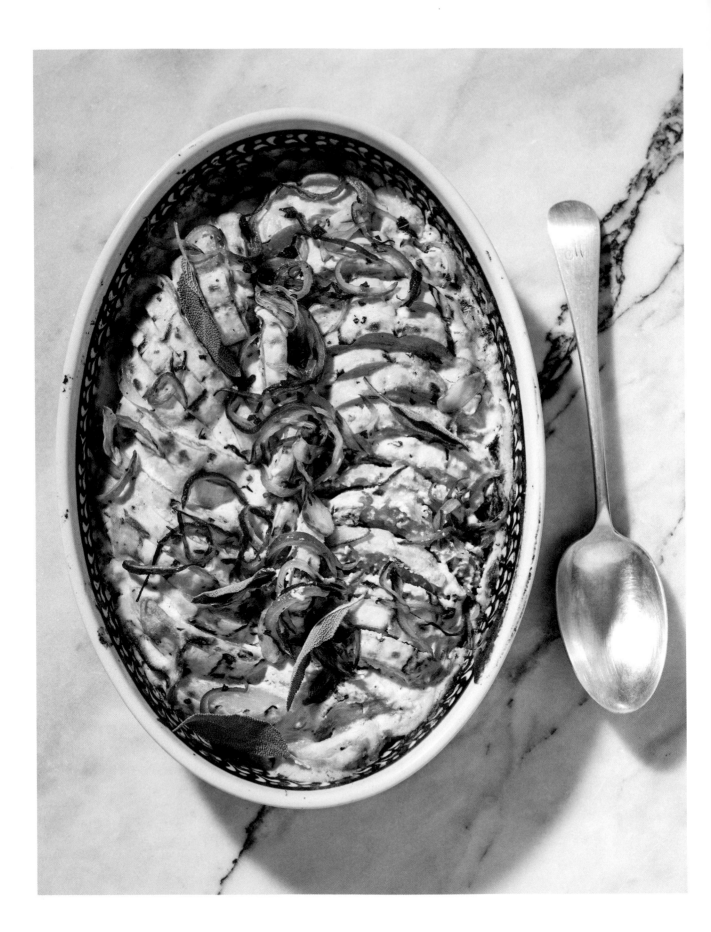

Squash Gratin with Cashew Cream

SERVES 6 TO 8

1 tablespoon plus 2 teaspoons olive oil, divided

1 large red onion, peeled and thinly sliced lengthwise

4 cloves garlic, peeled and thinly sliced

2 tablespoons coarsely chopped sage

Kosher salt and freshly ground black pepper

1 cup unsweetened almond milk

½ cup Cashew Cream Dressing (page 205)

2 tablespoons (packed) fresh thyme leaves, lightly chopped

½ teaspoon ground nutmeg

2 medium delicata squash (2 pounds), halved, seeded, and cut crosswise into ½-inch half-moons

I love the idea of a gratin anything—cheesy, gooey, warm—that is so my happy place. And when I get that craving, but I am trying to take a break from all the cheese and cream and milk, we make this recipe. Cashew cream is a great base substitute for a lot of creamy recipes, and we use it often at the house (think béchamel or cream sauces, and dressings like vegan ranch or Caesar).

There are a lot of sweet notes in the recipe from the squash, the almond milk, and the onions, so I really like to amp up the freshly ground black pepper. With the yummy sage and a dash of nutmeg, this dish screams fall.

Preheat oven to 400 degrees.

Make the cream sauce. Heat a medium skillet over medium-high heat. Add 1 tablespoon olive oil and swirl to coat. Add the onions, garlic, and sage and season with ½ teaspoon each salt and pepper. Sauté, stirring, until the onions are softened and begin to turn golden brown, about 6 minutes, reducing the heat as necessary to prevent burning. Remove the pan from the heat. Add the almond milk, Cashew Cream Dressing, thyme, and nutmeg. Stir until smooth and season to taste with more pepper.

Assemble the gratin. Lightly grease a broiler-safe 9-inch cake pan or casserole dish with the remaining 2 teaspoons olive oil. Working from the outside of the pan in, place one layer of squash in the pan, shingling the pieces in a circular fashion. Season with ½ teaspoon of salt and a generous pinch of pepper. Pour a third of the cream sauce over the squash, spreading with a small spatula to make sure that all the pieces are covered. Repeat, alternating layers of squash and cream sauce, finishing with the cream sauce on top (3 layers total of each).

Bake. Transfer the prepared gratin to the oven. Bake for 40 to 45 minutes, rotating halfway through, until the squash is tender and golden on the edges and the cream sauce is set.

For an extra crisp. Turn the broiler on high and broil, watching carefully to avoid burning. Broil until the top of the gratin is browned and crisp, 1 to 2 minutes. Remove from the oven and serve.

SIDES

GREENOA WITH CHARRED ROMAINE PESTO | *see page 207*

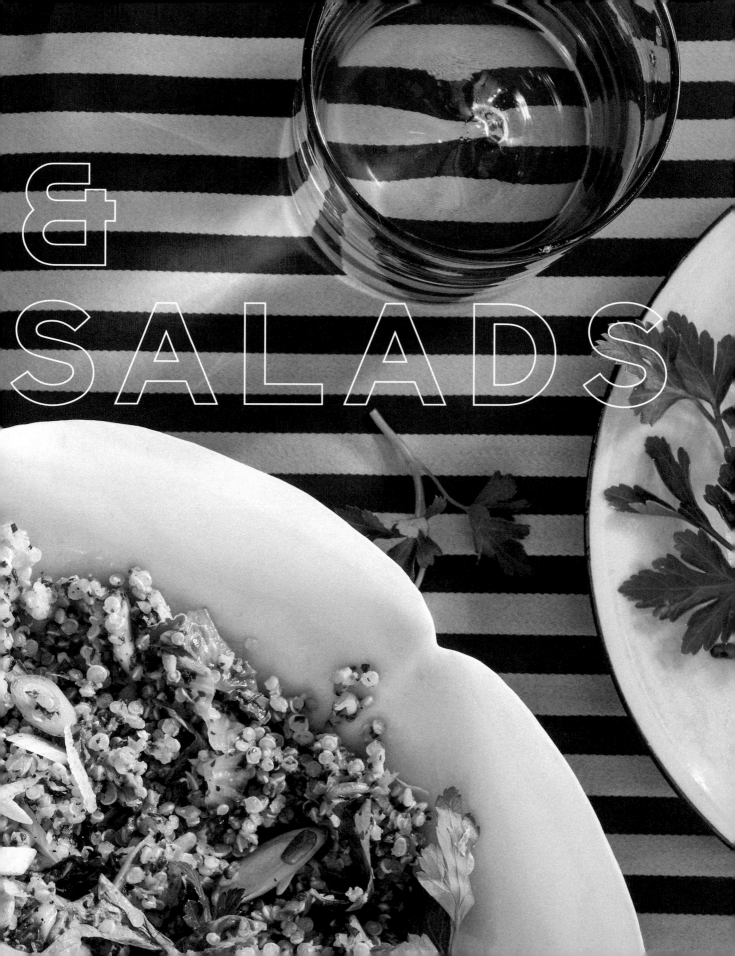

& SALADS

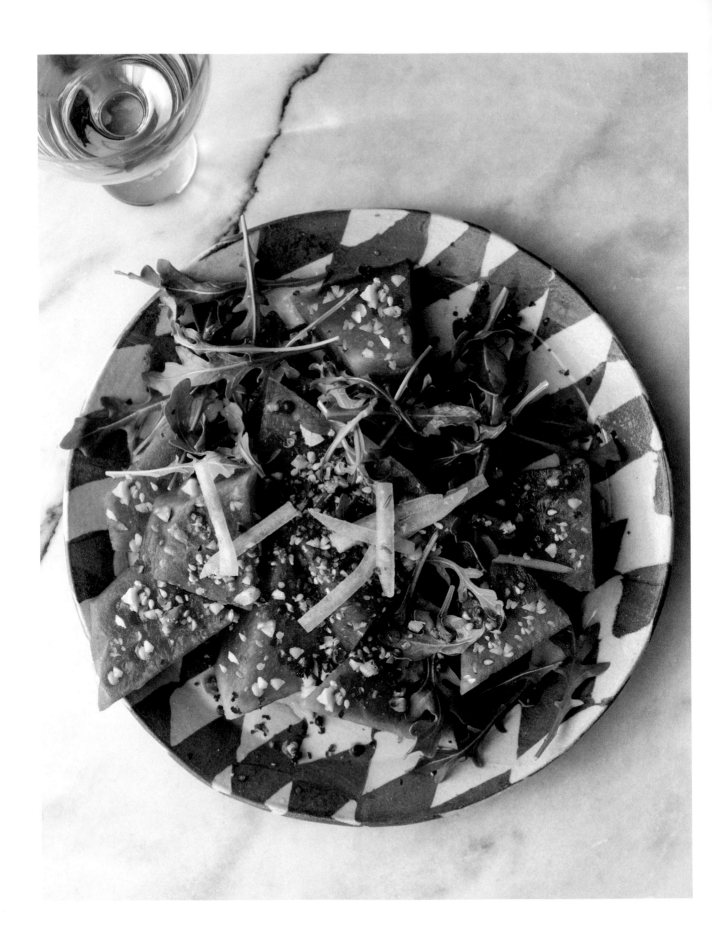

Watermelon with Pistachio Dukkah

SERVES 2 TO 4

½ baby, seedless watermelon, peeled, white rind reserved; flesh cut into irregular 2-inch pieces (about 4 to 5 chunks per person), chilled

¾ cup water

¾ cup apple cider vinegar

1 tablespoon plus 1 teaspoon honey, divided

½ teaspoon fennel seed

1½ teaspoons coriander seed, divided

1¼ teaspoons cumin seed, divided

Kosher salt and freshly ground black pepper

¾ teaspoon crushed pink peppercorns, divided

2 tablespoons sesame seeds

½ cup shelled pistachios, hazelnuts, or a mix of both, toasted and finely chopped, with some slightly larger pieces remaining

1 tablespoon hemp seeds

Flaky sea salt (we love Maldon)

1½ tablespoons olive oil

2 teaspoons freshly squeezed lemon juice

2 heaping cups baby arugula

This might be one of the first recipes we worked on for this book, and it still remains one of my favorites.

Dukkah is an Egyptian spice–nut blend that is super versatile—it can be used as a seasoning (pretty killer on popcorn), as a dip with some olive oil and bread, or in this case as a topping to fresh watermelon.

We love being able to use up all the different parts of the watermelon, so we make a quick pickle with the rind, which is both delicious and fun!

The dukkah and the pickled watermelon rind can be made in advance. It's one of my favorite salads, and makes a great snack, too. We hope you enjoy!

Make the quick-pickled watermelon rinds. Dice the watermelon rinds into ¼-inch cubes until it measures 1 cup (about 5 ounces). Place in a small heat-proof bowl.

Combine the water, apple cider vinegar, 1 tablespoon honey, fennel seed, ½ teaspoon coriander seed, ½ teaspoon cumin seed, 2 teaspoons kosher salt, and ½ teaspoon pink peppercorns in a small pot. Place over medium-high heat and bring to a bare simmer, stirring, until the salt and honey are dissolved. Pour over the watermelon rinds and let pickle, for 30 minutes in advance. Keep refrigerated until ready to use. (Leftover pickled watermelon rinds can be stored in an airtight container in the refrigerator for up to 1 week.)

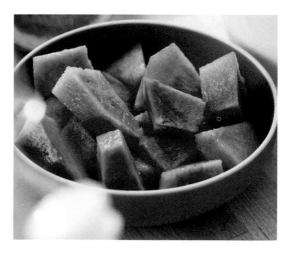

Make the dukkah. Combine the remaining 1 teaspoon coriander seed and ¾ teaspoon cumin seed in a small skillet. Place over medium heat and toast, shaking the pan occasionally, until somewhat darkened and fragrant, 2 to 3 minutes. Transfer to a mortar and pestle or spice grinder and grind until fine. Transfer the toasted spices to a small bowl. To the same skillet, add the sesame seeds and toast until lightly golden, shaking the pan, 1 to 2 minutes. Transfer to the bowl with spices. Add the nuts, hemp seeds, 1½ teaspoons flaky sea salt, remaining ¼ teaspoon pink peppercorns, and ¼ teaspoon black pepper. Mix to combine. Dukkah can be made ahead and kept at room temperature, in an airtight container, for up to 1 month.

Make the salad dressing. Combine the olive oil, lemon juice, and remaining 1 teaspoon honey. Whisk to emulsify. Season to taste with salt and pepper.

To assemble. Lightly toss the arugula in the dressing and divide among serving plates. Dip the watermelon pieces in the dukkah and place on top of the arugula. Garnish with pickled watermelon rinds and serve with additional dukkah, if desired.

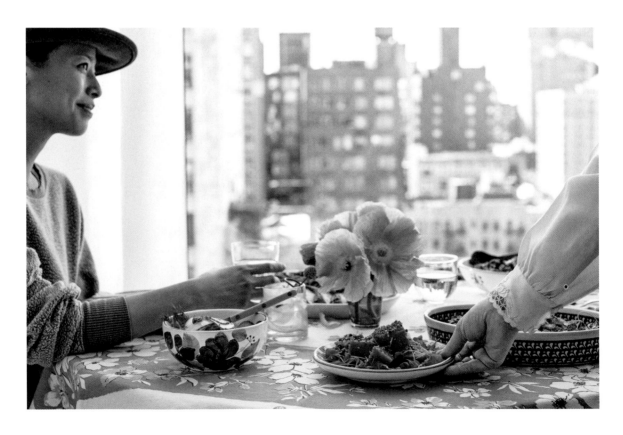

Cashew Cream Dressing

2 cups raw cashews (about ½ pound)

1 cup warm water

2 tablespoons dijon mustard

2 tablespoons apple cider vinegar

2 tablespoons white miso paste

Kosher salt and freshly ground black pepper

This cashew cream recipe makes a wonderful dairy substitute, and we use it in our Squash Gratin (page 199) and a variation of it in our vegan version of Pasta al Limone with Peas (page 180). It also works great as a creamy base for dressings like a vegan ranch or vegan Caesar. We like to whip up a batch and use it in different recipes throughout the week.

Soak your cashews. Place the cashews in a small bowl and add just enough water to cover. Let sit, at least 1 hour at room temperature or up to 2 days, covered, in the refrigerator.

Blend. Drain the cashews and rinse. Combine the cashews, warm water, dijon mustard, apple cider vinegar, and miso paste in a blender. (An immersion blender also works!) Blend until the mixture is very smooth and creamy with no grainy bits remaining, scraping down the sides of the bowl as necessary. Season with salt and pepper to taste. Cashew cream can keep, covered, in the refrigerator, for up to 5 days.

Cumin-Scented Slaw

MAKES 3 HEAPING CUPS
SERVES 2 TO 4

3 cups (lightly packed and heaping) shredded red and/or green cabbage

Kosher salt and freshly ground black pepper

2 teaspoons cumin seeds

2 tablespoons freshly squeezed lemon juice

½ tablespoon honey

1 to 2 teaspoons harissa paste, depending on desired heat level

1½ teaspoons mayonnaise of choice (we keep it vegan and use Vegenaise)

1 cup shredded carrots

2 stalks celery, peeled and cut crosswise, into ½-inch pieces

1 scallion, thinly sliced, white and green parts separated

I'm a coleslaw girl and nothing makes me happier. I like to have it in the fridge and snack on it throughout the day.

Pilar added a little spin on the classic coleslaw, by dialing back the mayonnaise and adding cumin and harissa—giving it a warm, slightly spicy layer of flavor. Harissa is truly one of my favorite condiments and I think it will be yours, too! It's originally from Tunisia and is made with a blend of dried chili peppers and olive oil, and some added seasonings. It's sooo delicious and gives dishes that extra-special oomph. (It can be found at most grocery stores and is easily available online, too!) Feel free to use your mayonnaise of choice; we use a vegan mayonnaise here to make the whole dish vegan, but regular mayonnaise would work as well.

Salt the cabbage. Salting your cabbage beforehand ensures that it remains crisp by removing excess moisture. Place the cabbage in a large bowl. Season with 1 teaspoon salt and toss to combine. Let it sit at room temperature, 10 to 20 minutes. Wrap the cabbage in paper towels or a clean kitchen cloth and squeeze to remove excess moisture. Return the cabbage to the bowl.

Make the dressing. Meanwhile, add the cumin seeds to a small skillet and place over medium heat. Toast, shaking the pan occasionally, until fragrant and toasted, 1 to 2 minutes. Let cool. Transfer to a small bowl. Add the lemon juice, honey, harissa paste, and mayonnaise. Whisk to combine and season to taste with salt and pepper.

Finish the slaw. Add the carrots, celery, and scallion whites to the bowl with the cabbage. Toss with the dressing until thoroughly coated. Season to taste with salt and pepper and let sit at least 20 minutes in the refrigerator, until chilled, and up to 2 hours in advance. Serve, garnished with scallion greens.

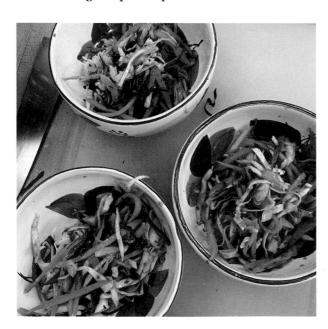

2 romaine hearts (about
  12 ounces), cut in half
  lengthwise

Kosher salt and freshly
  ground black pepper

2 teaspoons olive oil, plus
  additional for serving

2¼ cups water, divided

1 small bunch flat-leaf spinach
  (5 ounces), tough stems
  removed, rinsed

1 tablespoon nutritional yeast
  (optional)

½ cup toasted blanched
  almond slivers, divided

1 cup white quinoa

½ cup toasted sunflower
  seeds

2 tablespoons freshly
  squeezed lemon juice, plus
  zest of 1 lemon

2 scallions, green and
  white parts, thinly sliced
  crosswise

¼ cup (packed) coarsely
  chopped cilantro

¼ cup (packed) coarsely
  chopped flat-leaf parsley

Greenoa with Charred Romaine Pesto

If you're looking to up your quinoa game, have I got a recipe for you.

There's a whole science to why we crave and are drawn to crunchy, crispy food. And you may have noticed from the recipes that I love a good, fresh crunch—celery, cucumbers, iceberg and romaine lettuce, bell peppers—and this recipe really delivers on that front.

Our greenoa has tons of texture and herbs, which makes for a very satisfying meal. Pilar loves the flavor of grilled lettuce and cabbage. The trick to it is making sure that you get a good char on one side of the romaine, which will give a toasty, nutty flavor, but also making sure that the rest of the wedge remains cool and raw, for texture. (And yes, the recipe can absolutely be made with precooked quinoa.) The charred romaine pesto is a departure from a traditional pesto, and we hope it will become a classic in your kitchen.

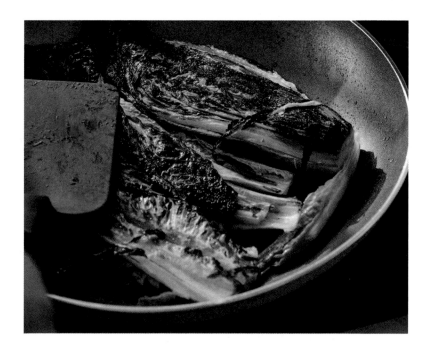

Make the romaine pesto. Heat a large skillet over high heat. Season the cut sides of romaine with salt and pepper, and drizzle with olive oil. Add to the hot skillet, cut-side down. Using a spatula, press down on the romaine slices until lightly charred but still crisp and raw on the outer layers, 1 to 2 minutes. Transfer to a cutting board and roughly chop. In a food processor, add half of the charred romaine, ¼ cup water, the spinach, nutritional yeast (if using), and ¼ cup of the almonds. Process until combined, scraping down the side of the food processor as necessary, until the mixture is finely chopped and resembles pesto. Season to taste with salt and pepper.

Make the quinoa. Place a medium pot over medium heat. Add the quinoa and a pinch of salt and toast, stirring frequently, until the quinoa is fragrant and a hue darker, about 2 minutes. Remove the pot from the heat and very slowly pour in the remaining 2 cups of water, being very careful as it will spatter. Return to heat and bring to a boil. Cover and reduce the heat to the lowest setting and simmer for 15 minutes. Remove from the heat and allow to steam, with the lid on, for an additional 5 minutes. Fluff the quinoa with a fork and transfer to a large bowl. Allow to cool to room temperature.

Serve. Pour the romaine pesto over the quinoa. Add the sunflower seeds, lemon zest and juice, scallions, cilantro, parsley, remaining almonds, and the reserved chopped romaine. Toss to combine and season to taste with salt and pepper and a drizzle of olive oil, if desired.

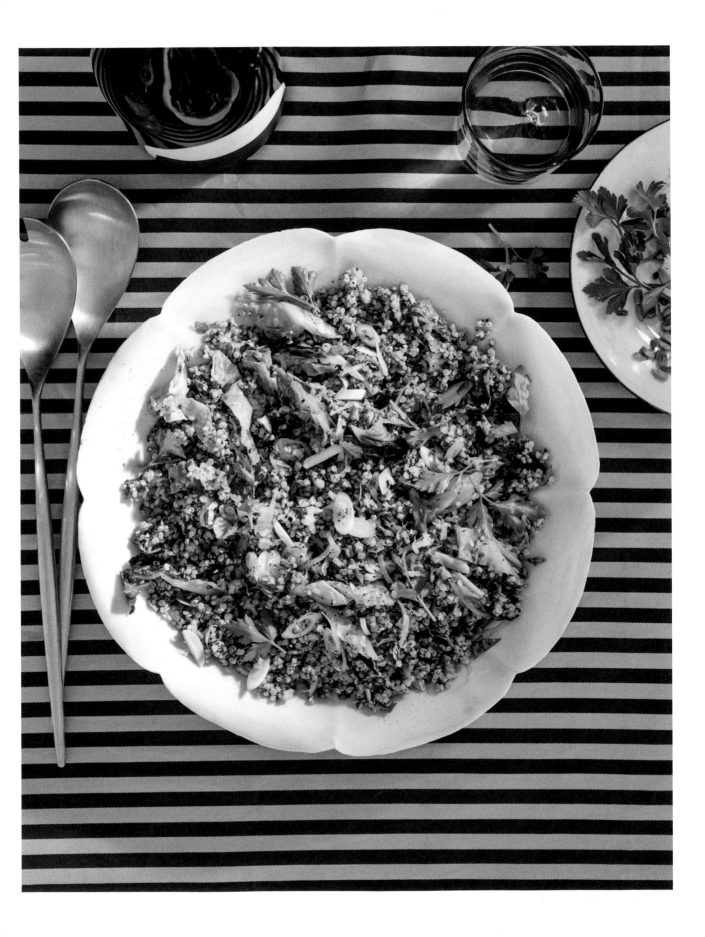

Light as Air Cuke Salad

MAKES ABOUT
2 HEAPING CUPS

SERVES 4 AS A SIDE

1 tablespoon vegan
  mayonnaise (we love
  Vegenaise)

1 tablespoon apple cider
  vinegar

Juice of ½ lemon

½ teaspoon honey

2 tablespoons (packed)
  drained and coarsely
  chopped capers, plus
  1 tablespoon caper brine

1 clove garlic, peeled and
  thinly sliced

2 teaspoons olive oil

3 tablespoons (packed)
  finely chopped dill, plus
  additional for serving

Kosher salt and freshly
  ground black pepper

1 English cucumber, thinly
  sliced crosswise

Flaky sea salt (we love
  Maldon), for serving

I adore this recipe because it is dead simple to make, and it hits all these different flavors—a li'l salty, li'l sweet, and li'l sour—combined with the fresh, crisp crunch of the cucumber. Yum.

One of Pilar's tips for using ingredients that are packed with brine (like capers, olives, hearts of palm, artichokes, etc.) is to use some of that brine in the dressing you make. It really adds that extra layer of flavor.

We love to use fresh herbs, and in this salad, the dill really shines. Feel free to use your mayonnaise of choice; we use a vegan mayonnaise here to keep it vegan, but regular mayonnaise would work, too. All the other ingredients are probably kicking around your pantry, making it an easy, go-to side salad recipe, perfect with any meal.

Make the dressing. In a large bowl, combine the mayonnaise, apple cider vinegar, lemon juice, honey, capers, caper brine, garlic, olive oil, and dill. Whisk to incorporate and season to taste with salt and pepper.

Add the cucumbers to the bowl and toss to coat. Let sit at least 1 hour in the refrigerator before serving.

Serve. Garnish with additional dill and flaky sea salt. Serve chilled.

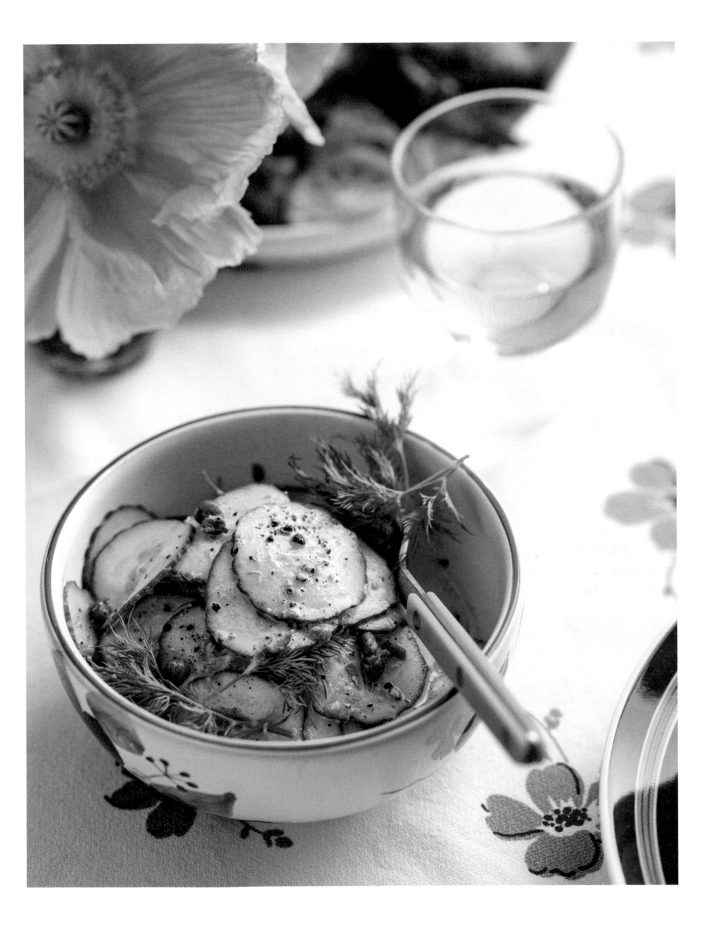

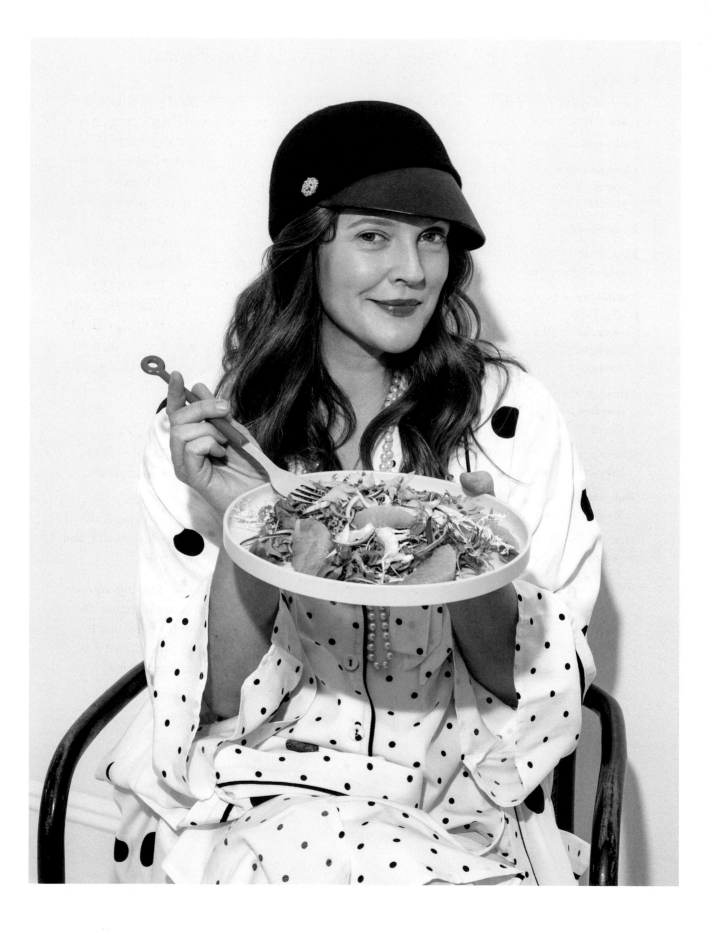

Pairs with Everything Salad

SERVES 4

¼ small red onion, thinly
sliced lengthwise

1 tablespoon balsamic vinegar

1 teaspoon orange blossom
honey (or substitute with
your favorite honey)

2 tablespoons olive oil

Kosher salt and freshly
ground black pepper

2 stalks celery, peeled and
sliced into ½-inch pieces
crosswise, leaves reserved
and lightly chopped, for
serving

1 small head (2 ounces) frisée,
trimmed and cut into 2-inch
pieces

2 heaping cups (1 ounce)
baby arugula

Flaky sea salt (we love
Maldon), for serving

1 navel or Cara Cara orange,
peeled and segmented

My love for celery knows no bounds, and you'll notice it sneaking into recipes here and there. When using celery raw, Pilar recommends shaving it with a vegetable peeler first, to remove the stringy and tough outer layer.

The vinaigrette is super simple and, with its sweet tang, uses only a small handful of items that you probably already have in your pantry.

A quick note on building a salad with the vinaigrette already in the bowl: we recommend starting with the heaviest ingredient on the bottom (in this case, the celery) and then adding the lighter ingredients on top (finishing with the baby arugula). This way, when you toss the ingredients to mix, your delicate greens won't get too overdressed.

Quick and easy, this salad goes with so many things and dresses up any meal.

Prepare the onions. Place the red onion slices in a small bowl of ice water. Let sit while you make the dressing. The cold water makes the onions crisp and keeps them fresh. Drain and pat dry before using.

Make the dressing. In a large bowl (big enough to fit the salad), combine the balsamic vinegar, honey, olive oil, ½ teaspoon salt, and ¼ teaspoon pepper. Whisk vigorously until emulsified.

Assemble the salad. Into the large bowl with the dressing, add the celery, frisée, red onion, and arugula. (We recommend adding the ingredients to the bowl by weight in that order, to ensure that the more delicate arugula does not get overdressed.) Toss to coat, and season with flaky sea salt and pepper. Divide among serving plates, top with celery leaves and orange segments, and serve.

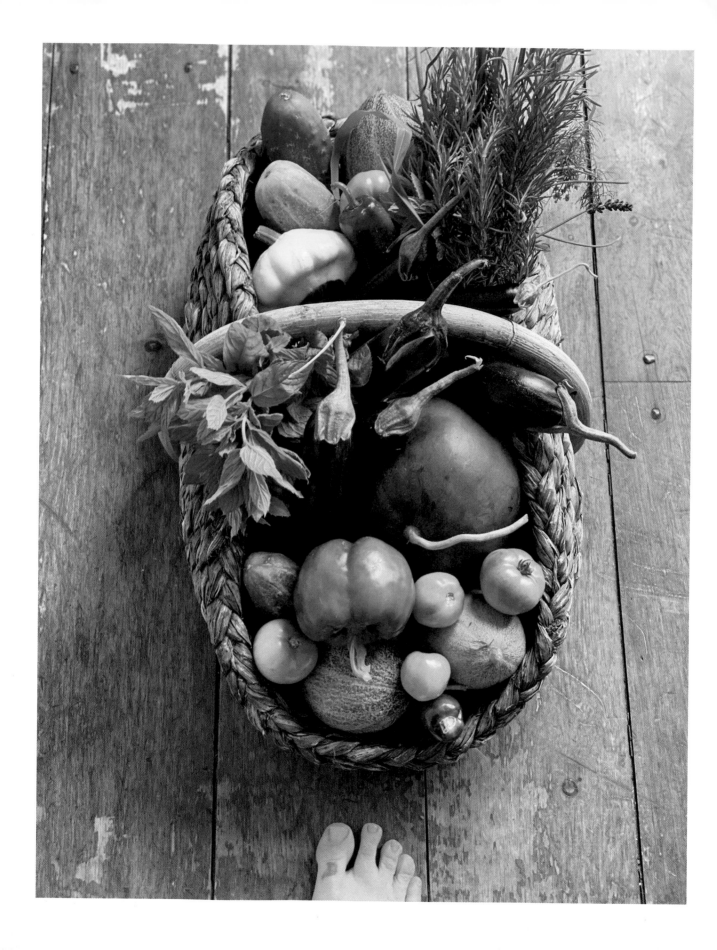

Evergreen

People say that life has many chapters, and it's tempting to think that its story is told in a neat, linear chronology, through the seasons that unfold predictably, year after year. But the tales that are actually told are far less predictable. Life goes up, down, and all around. Nature has regular cycles: winter becomes spring, then summer, and autumn, and nature is the most powerful thing. It's mighty, and we must bow down to it.

During the past year and a half, from winter 2020 to summer 2021, nature became the one thing I turned to for stability. Yes, nature has evolved, ice ages turning into hot, arid deserts where an ocean once stood. But for the most part, in a human life cycle, we can turn to nature for some type of predictability. The calendar is a broad map, and every autumn and winter, nature will hide and then finally fall into a slumber. But then, at last, spring comes, and things start to bloom. A bud of hope and a seed of change.

So many people know the cycles by heart. But I have lived my whole life in sunny California. And since 1975, I could rely on good weather 365 days a year. We might have the occasional rainy week, but that's about it. And we would welcome the rain, as smog would get rinsed away (and eventually creep back in). My dependable optimism is probably rooted in the "75 degrees and sunny" lifestyle that I was born, raised, and remained in until I moved to New York for my family, as I've mentioned earlier in this book.

Until I moved to the East Coast, my life had no seasons. But once the pandemic hit, I started to learn nature's cycles, then to crave them, and it saved me in many ways. For the first time in my life, I was able to look to nature and all its many forms within a cycle of a year, and it taught me and guided me through such an awful time of fear and uncertainty. Everything else felt scary, but nature was acting normal.

I've written about all the work I wanted to do, and was thrilled to do, in our new house. But I haven't shared how inspired I was by what was already there, and by all the things that inspired me! I felt it the first time during one of my walks in March 2020, when I found a tiny, bright yellow bud. It was called forsythia, and that was where my journey began. This tiny yellow birth gave me hope. It was a total kick-start to align my life with nature and have it teach me its ways. I was a student, and from there I would become a gardener. It felt perfect—I have always worked under the moniker FLOWER: Flower Films, Flower Beauty. And in Los Angeles, one takes for granted that flowers are always there. It's literally ever green! But here on the East Coast, an evergreen meant something else. I would learn the definition—and which species had lasted all winter, which would be there the next winter, and which would disappear.

I came to learn the Latin names of plants, and when one varietal bloomed and when another would take its bow. I created a symphony in this yard. I would learn the notes and sections. And so my peace was found walking around this yard, looking for the signs of spring, and the signs of hope. Like a green leaf popping up on a tree. I would take drives with the girls and put on an album for them, and as we drove (this felt like the huge break of our day), we would look at all the trees and fauna we could take in. *Hey, that one is blooming over there? In April? Okay, so things do come alive! And that's a cherry blossom, and that one is a dogwood. And they become green around May. Okay, got it. That is a Sango-kaku, a Japanese maple. It's red all year on its spinet base, but*

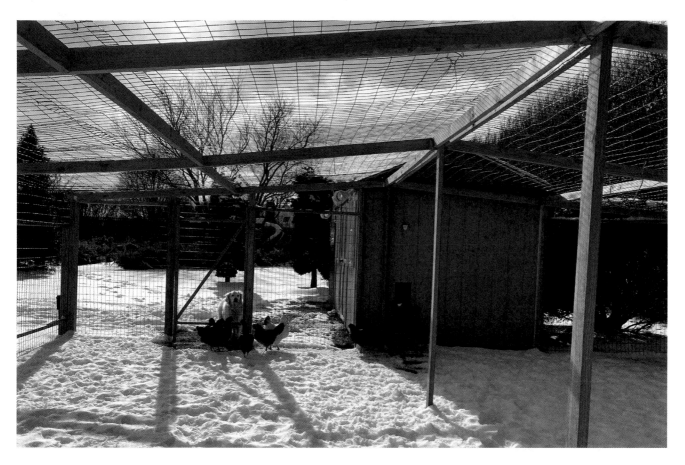

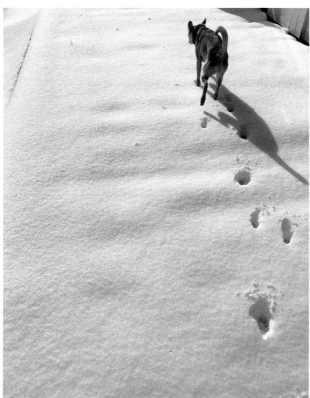

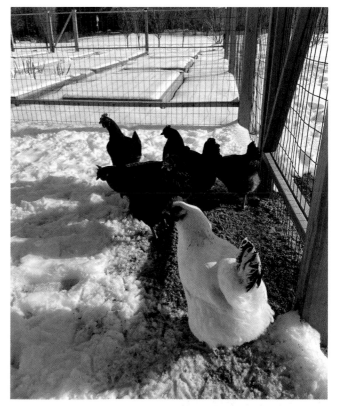

then come May to October, it has bright, light green leaves. Hornbeams. Nishikis. Rhodo-
dendron. Wisteria. Magnolias (crazy-short window; sneeze and you miss them!).

I started shopping trees for my future project—holy cow... not cheap. I would drive around and see people's yards and covet the old oaks that must have been there for hundreds of years. Or wonder if that abandoned parking lot needed that forsythia that was falling over and becoming weeds rather than being watered and loved (I can see it now, arrested for stealing trees). I began looking at each flower with purpose and a new curiosity.

Finally, I had been studying for months and I was ready to go. I went to the nursery with a big list. It was a daunting task creating the watercolor landscape I imagined. Midway through the conversation, Paige, the woman I was working with at the nursery, suggested I get a landscaper. She didn't think I had what it took to do this entire project as a whole. She said, "Why don't you come back when you have a plan."

And I looked at her in the eyes and said, "I'm doing this myself. We all have to rely on ourselves right now and this is going to be my project! I'm going to pour myself into this, and it's a spiritual endeavor. It's going to go piece by piece... So show me some fucking plants, please!" Her stern face turned into a wry smile. "I think I have exactly what you need. Let's get started!"

And with that we became wonderful friends. I mean, we spent the next year laughing. Picking out everything. I thought I couldn't have found a better teacher and companion. Paige was used to fussy people and loved that I was a rebel. Turns out she was one, too! She was into the fact that I didn't have cookie-cutter tastes, and her "wild garden style" (her actual account on Instagram!) was a perfect match for a rebel homemaker like me.

It took a while, but the trees arrived. I planted them, and everything was finally fully blooming, becoming summer. I also learned how to plant an entire fruit-and-veggie garden, something I could really sink my teeth into. Literally! Soon, I'd be able to eat actual food I had grown! And as things opened up little by little in the summer, I was ready! First in line with planting. First in line with my grass seed, throwing it all over the ground and watching my chickens grow. One day soon we would have eggs as well. The harvest would be in before we knew it.

I think one of the hardest parts when life is scary and gets turned upside down is to trust that things will heal. And to keep on trusting, even when you have no idea when that might happen. When will things be less scary? When will it not hurt so much? When will life stabilize? How do I deal with loss? Is it okay to be angry about loss? How do I deal with my range of emotions when I haven't been given an end date to any of this?

If there is an answer, it's patience, and the healing is up to me. Every life on this planet deals with birth, death, loss, fear, chaos, divorce, job loss, devastation, anxiety, tremendous backbreaking change with no reprieve in sight. None of us escapes all those things on this journey of life. And what was so amazing, through the pandemic, was everyone experiencing it at the exact same time. But just like in life, there were different scales and measurements. Sometimes nature reflects this, too. A tornado versus a rainstorm. The balance can seem utterly off, and with no ability to compare the impact.

But what I learned in this pandemic, and won't forget, was how looking to nature healed me. If it was acting normal, then maybe everything around it would return one day, too. As we all stayed frozen in time, I watched things go from asleep and seemingly gone forever into a small, tiny bloom of life. And then a roar of color!

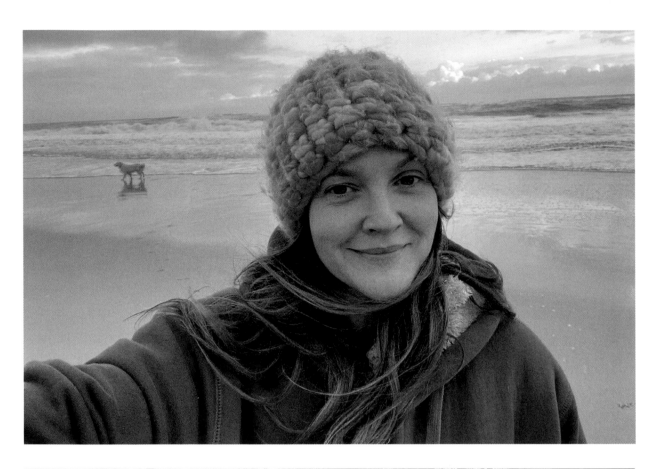

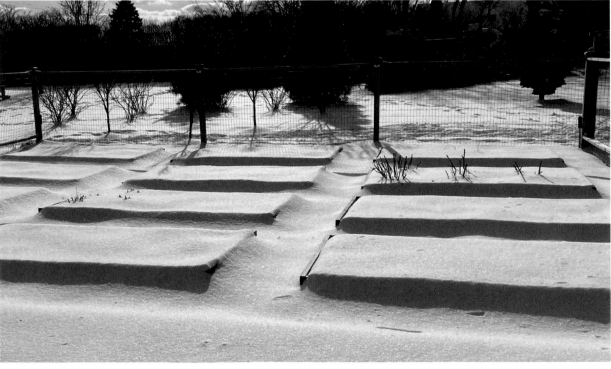

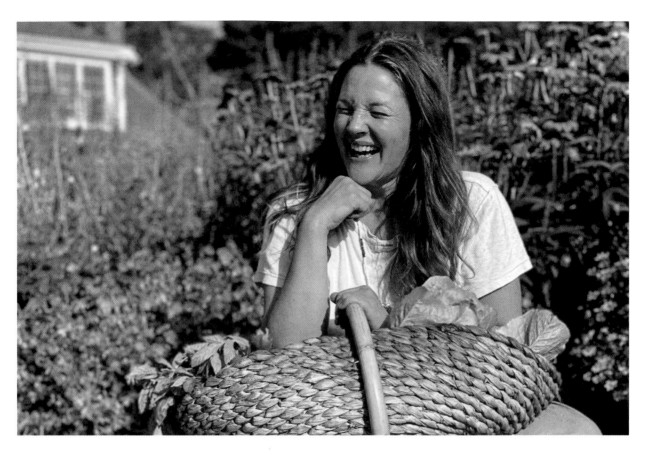

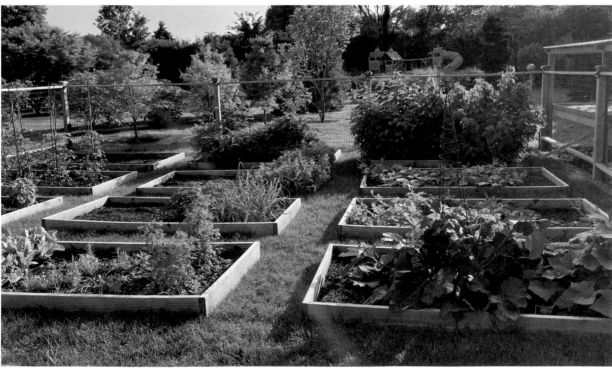

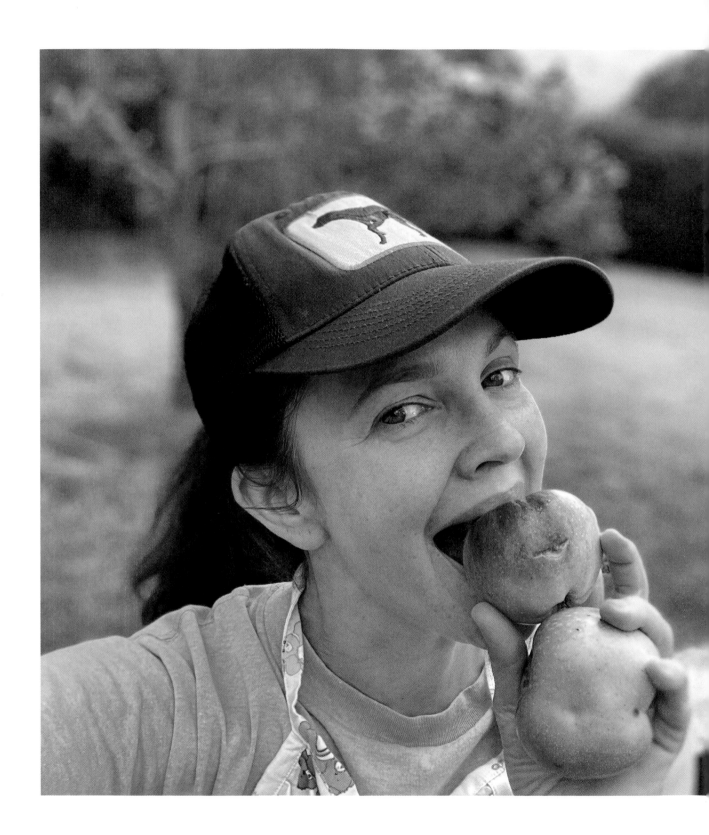

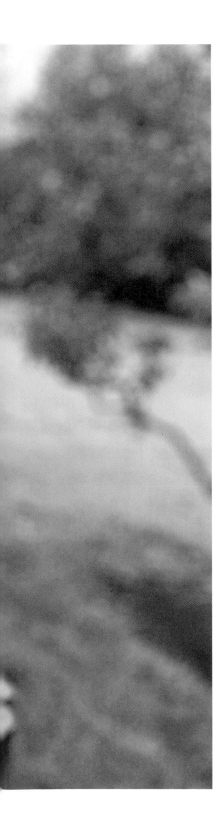

Life goes in cycles. As in nature. And we hold on tight. Trying to witness as much as we can. I look away and our kids are a year older, I've been doing this crazy talk show job for a year now, and all of a sudden, the tree outside has leaves. Blink and you could miss it. But if we are forced to *stop* and stare and wait, it all goes in slow motion, but it does come alive again. The cycle takes place and the roller coaster goes up and down . . . but it is a lovely, emotional, complex, and truly beautiful ride.

Acknowledgments

I would like to thank Jill Schwartzman! She is the best book editor because she is candid as well as enthusiastic. She ensures good and honest work to flow out of me. And our second collaboration has been another yearlong endeavor that was both thoughtful and personal. Jill, I love putting our heads and hearts together. I love getting to know you and work with you.

Pilar . . . it isn't enough to dedicate this book to you, I also need to say I just wouldn't be doing this without you. I love our test kitchen and how much we laugh out loud. But boy do we care! You would never know how much we cackle by how seriously we take our passions. But we do and here's to more . . .

Nora Singley, our fearless recipe developer. When COVID hit, you and Pilar became superheroes on Zoom and created the genius translation of all our flavor and culinary intentions! You made it real and you made it make sense. You are so important to this book, and through every decision you made, you helped us translate our world to others. Thank you so much.

Graydon Herriott! Thanks to your photography, we were able to make the book of our dreams, but you also let me integrate real life into it. You make everything look so amazing and beautiful. And yet it's also inspiring and aspirational. Thank you for letting me weave in my life along with your brilliance and joy!

Thanks to the whole team at Dutton who made this possible, especially John Parsley, who was able to truly help realize a unique vision for this book and was always someone we could truly rely on, and Lorie Pagnozzi, who executed everything with such a graphic and poetic eye. Thanks also to Christine Ball, Jamie Knapp, Stephanie Cooper, Katie Taylor, Tiffany Estreicher, LeeAnn Pemberton, Susan Schwartz, Dora Mak, Marya Pasciuto, Christopher Lin, and Vi-An Nguyen.

Thanks also to CAA, especially Mollie Glick, who literally helped this actually happen. She has been the true champion of this endeavor since day one. And here we are, Mollie . . . about to cross the finish line together.

Special thanks to everyone who I get to make *The Drew Barrymore Show* with. Our love of cookbook club and all the amazing food adventures we get to go on!! I am so excited to celebrate this with you. And let's keep exploring the world of food and the incredible chefs who make it.

Thank you, too, Ember Truesdell, Wilfredo Perdomo, Sidney Wertimer, Crystal Meers, Christy Doramus, Anna Golino, Francesca de la Fuente, Omar Lagda, and the whole team, my work family. With a very important thank-you, Naz Sahin and Joanna Bean Martin of AfterAll studio, for your endless exploration and incredible inspiration on how to make this cover come alive! You all truly helped me make this book while trying to juggle it all like a lunatic. You are all what makes everything I ever dream to do actually possible. Thank you for being such incredible humans.

Chris Miller. Best partner. Best person. And thank you for helping me take this on, along with everything else we try to do. I love doing it with you. My trusted brother.

To Olive and Frankie . . . you are my reason for everything I do and care about. You are my universe. And I love you more than all the words in all the books.

Credits

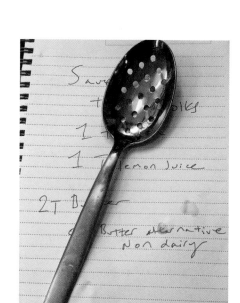

All recipes developed by Drew Barrymore and Pilar Valdes

Recipe writing and testing by Nora Singley

Additional recipe testing by Kristina Kurek

Photographers: Graydon Herriott

Food stylist: Eugene Jho

Set designer: Kalen Kaminski

Personal photographs courtesy of the author

Set design loans courtesy of the following friends and small businesses:

Ivy Ceramics: ivyivyivy.com

Laura Chautin Ceramics: laura-chautin.com/ceramics

Summer School Shop Ceramics: summerschoolshop.com/shop

Studio Iris Furniture: fleuroticaflowers.com

Upstate, Glassware: youreupstatecom.com

Herriott Grace, Wooden Spoons: herriottgrace.com

Index

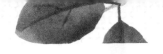
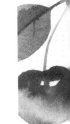

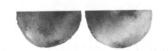

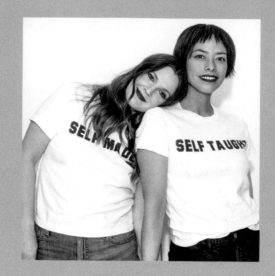

About the Authors

DREW BARRYMORE is a mother, actor, producer, entrepreneur, and *New York Times* bestselling author. She captured our hearts when she starred in *E.T.* at the age of six and has gone on to win critical acclaim for her work in movies such as *The Wedding Singer, Ever After, Charlie's Angels,* and *Grey Gardens,* to name a few. She is the host of *The Drew Barrymore Show,* as well as the founder of Flower Films, Flower Beauty, and the kitchen brand Beautiful.

PILAR VALDES was born and braised in the sticky tropical hearth of Manila, Philippines, amid the spin of her family's lazy Susan. She graduated with a BA from Sarah Lawrence College and spent the early years of her professional life working with young people through popular education workshops and video storytelling. In 2010, longing for both the proverbial stove of her childhood and relationships forged over shared meals, she switched careers and co-founded Kickshaw Cookery, a bespoke catering company placing a premium on carefully sourced ingredients and thoughtfully crafted menus. She currently works as a private chef and is a regular culinary contributor on *The Drew Barrymore Show.* She has always been a good eater.